Apple Cider Vinegar and Coconut Oil For Weight Loss

2-in-1 Secret Essential Oil And Successful Natural Remedy For Faster Weight Loss Boxed Set

Jessica David

Includes:

Apple Cider Vinegar
For Weight Loss

The Secret Of A Successful Natural Remedy
For Faster Weight Loss

&

Coconut Oil For Weight Loss

The Secret Of An Ancient Essential Oil
For Faster Weight Loss

APPLE CIDER VINEGAR
FOR WEIGHT LOSS

The Secret Of A Successful Natural Remedy For Faster Weight Loss

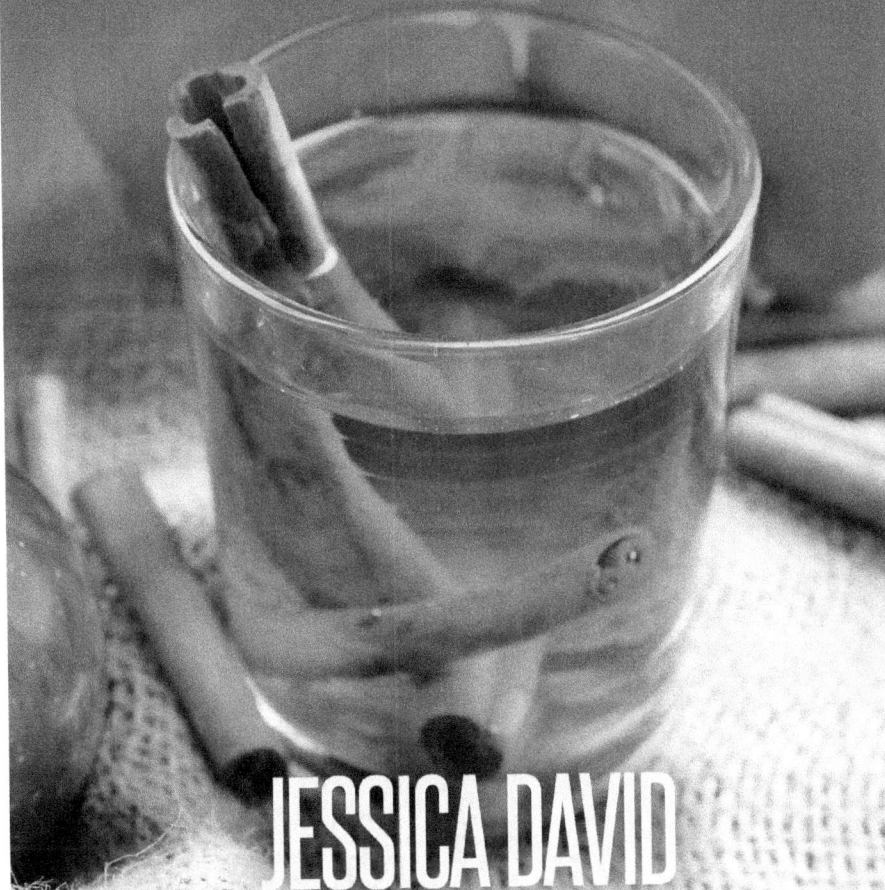

JESSICA DAVID

Book 1: Apple Cider Vinegar For Weight Loss

The Secret Of A Successful Natural Remedy For Faster Weight Loss

Jessica David

COPYRIGHT

Copyright © 2015

DISCLAIMER

Your Free Gift

As a special Thank You for downloading this book I have put together an exclusive report on "Superfoods For Weight Loss".

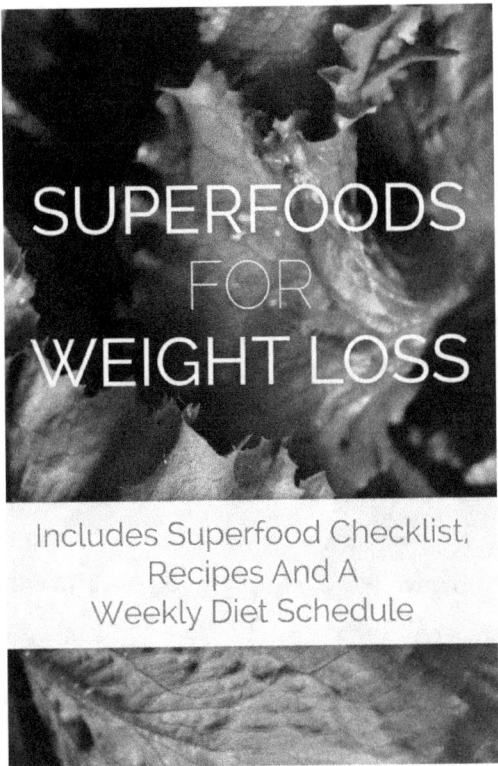

Learn about simple superfoods that can not only help you los weight but also, strengthen your body and improve mental performance. These foods are packed with nutrients, antioxidants and often have amazing side bonuses – like cancer fighting agents. Includes a superfood checklist and an easy to follow diet schedule.

>> You Can Download This Free Report By Clicking Here <<

FREE GIFT

Kindle 5 Star Books

Free Kindle 5 Star Book Club Membership

Join Other Kindle 5 Star Members Who Are Getting Private Access To Weekly Free Kindle Book Promotions

Get free Kindle books

Stay connected:

Join our Facebook group

Follow Kindle 5 Star on Twitter

Also, if you want to receive updates on Jessica David's new books, free promotions and Kindle countdown deals sign up to her New Release Mailing List.

TABLE OF CONTENTS

INTRODUCTION

Traditionally, apple cider vinegar was used in cooking to flavor and preserve food. Vinegar has been used as a folk remedy for many years for various ailments such as warts, the flu, head lice and used along with honey as a remedy for persistent coughs.

In more recent years, apple cider vinegar, also called cider vinegar, has been studied scientifically to examine the health benefits it may provide. Some of this interest may come from the creation of vinegar drinks in Japan in the 2000s, which itself stemmed from the age-old use of vinegar to aid in health. This trend has now slowly migrated to the West. Such interest also stems from a 1958 book by a Vermont-based folk doctor name D.C. Jarvis. While the majority of herbalists, as well as the medical science establishment, have dismissed Jarvis' claims for improved health through apple cider vinegar consumption, in recent years there has been renewed interest in using apple cider vinegar for weight loss. This may perhaps be due to the current obesity problem in the US coupled with the current interest in seeking treatment for health problems outside of the realm of traditional medicine. Various studies have been performed on apple cider vinegar as well as other vinegars to determine their potential health benefits. Although much more research is needed to draw any strong conclusions about health benefits, as a functional food, vinegar — including apple cider vinegar — *may* benefit various part of the body, including the cardiovascular system and the brain. Additionally, vinegar has been shown to have other positive health effects, including the potential to aid in weight loss for overweight individuals. Again, there needs to be a lot more scientific research performed before the potential health benefits of vinegar can be more firmly established, and not all scientists and doctors agree that it can help you lose weight. Only a few studies have looked at the use of apple cider vinegar for weight loss; the sample size is simply too small to draw any solid scientific conclusions.

What follows is a discussion about vinegar, its traditional uses and what scientific research says about its potential health benefits. Since it is established as a food ingredient throughout the world to preserve food and give it flavor, recipes for food and drink that include apple cider vinegar as well as other vinegars are included. Lastly, various sources of information in order to find reliable data on natural medical products and treatments, including apple cider vinegar, are provided.

CHAPTER 1

Some Background on Apple
Cider and Other Vinegars

A Little History

The English word vinegar comes from the French phrase for "sour wine" or "vin aigre," as it is written in French. Vinegar has been utilized since ancient times to not only flavor and preserve food but also for medicinal purposes. The Greek doctor, Hippocrates, the father of modern medicine after whom the Hippocratic Oath is named, used vinegar as a wound treatment. He also suggested the use of a honey and vinegar mixture to treat persistent cough. Sung Tse, the Chinese 10th century inventor of forensic medicine, suggested using a mixture of sulfur and vinegar when washing hands to prevent infections during autopsies. Apple cider vinegar was used to treat pneumonia during the American Civil War and had been used by 18th century doctors in the US as a remedy for a variety of ailments such as edema (or dropsy as it was called then), poison ivy and stomach ache. During World War II, it was used to treat wounds. Samurai warriors used to consume vinegar in order to obtain power and vigor.

Vinegar is used around the world and can come in many forms. Apple cider vinegar is manufactured globally, but there are many other forms that are particular to a certain country. For instance, in Japan, Kurosu vinegar is made; in France and the US, champagne vinegar is manufactured. In Italy and Turkey, white wine vinegar is made. Below is a list of other types of vinegars and where they are made.

	Vinegar Type	Country of Manufacture
1	Red wine vinegar	Worldwide
2	Balsamic vinegar	Italy
3	Cane vinegar	Philippines
4	Beer vinegar	Germany
5	Distilled vinegar	United States
6	Sherry vinegar	Spain
7	Potato vinegar	Japan
8	Spirit vinegar	Germany
9	White wine vinegar	Italy, Turkey
10	Tarragon vinegar	United States
11	Malt vinegar	England
12	Coconut vinegar	Southeast Asia
13	Fruit vinegar	Austria

How Vinegar is Made

Vinegar can come in a variety of flavors since it can be produced by nearly any "fermentable carbohydrate source," such as fruit (apples, plums, berries, etc.), beer, malt, whey, honey, coconuts, and grains, among other sources.

It can be made at home or on an industrial scale. In the home-made version of apple cider vinegar, some starter materials like apple cores and peels from organic apples, are placed in a sterile, wide-mouth, large jar. Then water is added (enough to cover the apple cores and skins in the jar). Some honey and one tablespoon of unpasteurized apple cider vinegar is added to start the fermentation process. The apple cider vinegar needs to be unpasteurized because the heating process called pasteurization kills the microorganisms needed to create the vinegar. The jar is covered with a paper towel and secured with a rubber band or metal jar ring; it is allowed to sit for two weeks in a cool, dark location. (Some recipes call for use of cheese cloth rather than a paper towel. However, the fruit flies that appear when using this cloth may lay their eggs in the vinegar, so avoiding cheese cloth is desirable.) After the two weeks, the liquid is strained and returned to the jar with the "mother" added to it. The mother is a grayish, white mass that is used in creating vinegar. This can be obtained from a jar of unpasteurized vinegar, like Bragg's Apple Cider Vinegar. It is then allowed to sit for four weeks with a new paper towel covering. The mixture is stirred daily. After the four weeks, the vinegar can be tasted to see if it has reached the desired level of acidity. If not, then it can be kept in the jar and checked every few days. To get a more mellow flavor, the vinegar can be poured out into clean jars separated from the scoby-which stands for symbiotic culture of bacteria and yeasts. (The scoby forms during fermentation.) The vinegar can then be capped and allowed to age for a few months.

Vinegar can be made on an industrial scale. The concept of industrial manufacturing of vinegar was first developed in 1823 by the German chemist Schutzenbach. Using his method vinegar could be made in 3 to 7 days. In 1955, Hromatka had created the submerged acedification method, which allowed for faster production of vinegar, by improving stirring and aeration. Just like homemade vinegar, industrial-made vinegar first goes through a fermentation process, in which ethanol is created. (When making apple cider vinegar at home, hard cider is made at this stage.) Next, it goes through a second fermentation stage in which acetic acid, the main ingredient in vinegar, is made from ethanol (drinking alcohol).

The surface method of production and the submerged culture method may be used to make vinegar on an industrial scale. In the surface method-often used for traditional vinegars-the acetic acid bacteria is present on the surface of the wood chips and supplies oxygen that this location. In the submerged method of vinegar creation, oxygen is added during fermentation to increase production. Industrial vinegars are often made using the generator method, which involves the use of large wooden vats. These vats contain filling made from either charcoal, grape pulp or beechwood chips that have been dipped in vinegar. Alcohol product is added to the vats and the alcohol moves through the fillings. Oxygen is added to the process via holes at the bottom of the vats and on their sides. By the time the liquid has moved through the fillings and reached the bottom of the vats, it has turned to a highly acidic form of vinegar that is at 14% acetic acid. To get the product to 5-6% acetic acid, dilution is needed. The typical household vinegar is 5% acetic acid. This is important, as contact with high concentrations of acetic acid in vinegar can be very harmful, harming the skin and eyes.

Balsamic vinegar is made in yet another way. For vinegar to be called traditional balsamic vinegar, it needs to be made from the Lambrusco or Trebbiano grapes grown in Emilia-Romagna region of Italy, in the northern part of the country. The must of the grapes (which includes the pips, skins and juice left over from wine pressing) are used to make this sort of vinegar. The juice is separated from the skins and seeds, filtered and boiled over an open flame for 24-30 hours. The liquid is carefully reduced to about 1/3 of its original size. It is then supplied with the "mother." The vinegar is then placed in wooded barrels which are then put in a warm location like an attic traditionally, and periodically are transferred new barrels. This is done over a period of 12 years (at minimum) at the end of which the liquid has been reduced from an initial volume of about 18 gallons to a volume of less than a gallon.

The French Orleans method of vinegar production is another traditional method. This technique may also be called the continuous method of vinegar making as it consists of juice being continuously added to barrels over a period of months. The barrels with holes in them are laid on their sides and filled with alcohol using a funnel. The mother is placed into the barrels as well. Some protective screens or netting are placed on the holes to prevent insects from getting inside. The barrels sit at a temperature of 85 degrees Fahrenheit or 29 degree Celsius. The product is removed from the barrel and about 15% is left in order to start the next batch of vinegar.

In Spain, the Philippines and other countries, there are other unique ways to make vinegar. Vinegar manufacturing is a time-honored tradition in various places around the world and most likely will continue to be so for years to come. Many health claims have been associated with vinegar use. As science has relatively recently started to investigate these claims, only some initial conclusions can be drawn, but much of it has been positive so far.

CHAPTER 2

Trying to Determine the "Secret" to Apple Cider Vinegar and Weight Loss or other Health Benefits

Some research studies have explored the potential health benefits of vinegar consumption. From these studies, it has been shown that vinegar, including apple cider vinegar, appears to have a positive impact on the body in many ways, including an anti-obesity and anti-oxidant effect. Consuming vinegar may also work against tumors, lower cholesterol, reduce high blood pressure, as well as work against bacterial infections, among several other health benefits. However, much more research needs to be done to make these results more conclusive.

Anti-Obesity Effects of Vinegar

Studies in Humans

A 2009 study in Japan looked at the use of apple cider vinegar for losing weight. Subjects in the experimental group were given apple cider vinegar while those in the control group consumed water. The study lasted for 12 weeks and included 175 obese people who were otherwise healthy. The subjects ate similar foods, but at the end of the 12 weeks the experimental group had lost more pounds than the control group, an average of 1-2 pounds. Researchers also found that the BMI (body mass index), serum triglyceride levels, visceral fat area and waist circumference were reduced in the group that consumed vinegar compared to the water group. The weight loss was not maintained after the conclusion of the study, however. The experimental group that took the apple cider vinegar gained their weight back. The study does help to illustrate that using this form of vinegar may help with weight loss. More research is required, however, before any conclusions can be made regarding the use of this type of vinegar for weight loss.

Numerous other studies have looked at the use of various types of vinegars and the potential weight loss benefits they may provide. Research by Johnson observed that subjects who daily consumed 2 tablespoons of red raspberry vinegar over a period of 4 weeks and who were free to eat and drink lost weight. In contrast, the control group who consumed 2 tablespoons of cranberry juice instead of vinegar, experienced slight weight gain during those 4 weeks. In a study by Mermel, it was stated that ingesting vinegar may reduce the glycemic effect of food consumption, thus leading a person to feel satisfied after eating. In other words, when someone consumes vinegar the change in blood sugar that comes from eating is reduced. This could potentially be of benefit for those with blood sugar problems like diabetics. Furthermore, in a 2005 experiment by Ostman and others, study subjects were provided with vinegar containing three levels of acetic acid, along with white wheat bread to consume. The control group only ate white wheat bread. At the study's conclusion, subjects who had the vinegar with the highest level of acetic acid reported the highest level of satiety. These and other studies seem to indicate that vinegar may assist in weight loss.

It is interesting to note that experiments with animals have yielded similar results. Budak and others observed that rats fed a high cholesterol diet and also given apple cider vinegar, had less steatosis (or fat in the liver) compared to the rats in the study not given this vinegar. In research by Lim and others, rats were given a type of vinegar made from Panax ginseng called Ginsam. In this study it was found that obese rats who were given this vinegar lost weight, and had more reduced plasma insulin levels and fasting, postprandial (after a meal) glucose levels compared to the controls.

Blood Pressure (Anti-hypertensive) Lowering Benefits

Vinegar may help with lowering blood pressure, or hypertension according to some studies. Although these studies were performed in rats, they may ultimately have benefit for people, but research would have to be performed in human subjects to make certain of this. Based on some of the research that so far has been performed, it appears that both the main component of vinegar, acetic acid, as well as other components found in some vinegar may help lower blood pressure. Research performed on rats by Nishikawa and others have shown that the residues from rice vinegar stop the activity of angiotensin-converting enzyme (ACE) in the system that regulates blood pressure. (Note: ACE, is a protein that gets converted from ACE I to ACE II in the body. The level of ACE increases or decreases based on the disease activity that the body is experiencing.) According to Rufian-Henares and Morales, melanoidins created in traditionally made balsamic vinegar lower blood pressure. Similar results were observed with acetic acid. In a study by, Honsho and others, used to test the anti-hypertensive effects of a Japanese vinegar and grape juice drink, ingestion of vinegar and acetic acid decreased the plasma level of the renin and the steroid aldosterone in rats. These biochemicals are associated with high blood pressure in rats.

Potential Benefits for Wounds

The components of vinegar may help in wound treatment. In a study by Sugiyama and others, dried acetic acid bacteria were given to study participants in the experimental group for a week. Those in the placebo group took an identical amount of corn starch. These participants then exercised for 60 minutes at the end of the week. The group that took the acetic acid, had less ankle pain, decreased neutrophil levels (neutrophils are white blood cells associated with inflammation in the body due to inflammation) and lower creatine kinase levels after exercising, compared to the placebo group. (Note: Creatine kinase is an enzyme associated with various conditions including muscle damage). Additionally, the mother (a mass of cells which forms from vinegar creation) appears to be able to help with burn treatment due to its anti-microbial effects. Also, acetobacter xylinum, an acetic acid bacterium that can be found in vinegars, like komesu used in Japan creates extracellular formations, which aid in tissue repair in rats.

Potential Benefits for the Brain

It has been suggested that vinegar may help with brain functioning in humans, according to Fukami and others. Moreover, the precursors of sphingolipids, called alkali-stable lipids can be produced by acetic acid bacteria. (Note: Sphingolipids are significant in the creation of brain tissue.) These alkali-stable lipids were seen to help rats with dementia greatly improve their cognition after day 10 of treatment with vinegar. Svennerholm found that gangliosides composed of certain molecules like sialic acid, improved symptoms of Alzheimer's disease.

Potential Benefits for the Cardiovascular System

High cholesterol, inactivity among other risk factors can lead to cardiovascular disease. Eating foods rich in polyphenols has been shown to reduce the chance of getting this condition. Apple cider vinegar has high levels of the polyphenol chlorogenic acid, which reduces low density lipoprotein, or LDL, (bad cholesterol) levels in the blood, according to Laranjinha and others. Other studies have shown the acetic acid lowers cholesterol and improved "lipid homeostasis." Additionally, a study by Budak and others observed that when rats had consumed apple cider vinegar created by the surface method with maceration their HDL (good cholesterol) levels were raised. Moreover, apple cider vinegar reduced the very low density lipoprotein (VLDL) and triglyceride levels in the rats in the experimental group. This was the case regardless of the vinegar's method of production. However, this type of vinegar also increased the LDL, HDL ad total cholesterol of the animals.

Certainly, more research needs to be performed to exactly determine the cholesterol-lowering abilities of apple cider vinegar.

Regular vinegar consumption may also help prevent ischemic heart attacks, based on a study by Hu and others. In this experiment, it was observed that those who had oil and vinegar salad dressing regularly, 5-6 times a week, had a greatly reduced risk of experiencing ischemic heart attacks, compared to those who ate creamy, mayonnaise-based dressings. It was hypothesized that the anti-arrhythmic component linolenic acid in the oil and vinegar salad dressings provided the heart benefit. Yet Johnson and Gaas noted that mayonnaise-based salad dressing also have lots of linolenic acid, so it might not be the reason for the reduction in ischemic heart attacks. However, perhaps there are other ingredients in the mayonnaise-based salad dressing, that are not present in the oil and vinegar-based dressings, that cancel out the benefits of the linolenic acid. More human clinical trials dealing with this issue need to be conducted to better understand the potential connection between linolenic acid intake and the risk of ischemic heart attacks.

Anti-tumor Benefits

Research by Mimura and others has shown that a Japanese vinegar made from sugar cane, called kibizu, can help to fight leukemia cells. Such vinegar also appeared to reduce the chance of getting esophageal cancer based on a study by Xibib and others. In this study the researchers looked at the incidence of esophageal cancer in Linzhou City in China, which has one of the highest rates of this form of cancer in the world. It was found that socio-economic status was closely linked to getting this disease. The poorer the person, the more likely they were to develop esophageal cancer. But study participants who consumed vinegar, vegetables and beans had a reduced risk of developing this cancer. Similarly, an ethyl acetate extract of a Japanese rice vinegar (Kurosu) seems to harm cancer cells. This anti-cancer effect was tested using various cells including lung carcinoma, colon adenocarcinoma, prostate cell carcinoma, breast adenocarcinoma, and bladder carcinoma. The vinegar inhibited the growth of cells for each cancer cell type. In another study, scientists gave an ethyl acetate extract of Kurosu to male rats with colon adenocarcinomas. (Adenocarcinomas describe cancers that form in the mucous membrane of the body.) After the animals were given a compound that induced the colon adenocarcinomas, they were given either water with the vinegar extract or water without the vinegar extract to drink. The animals given the water with the vinegar extract had smaller cancers than those who drank the water alone. These results are like those found in another study involving the use of rice vinegar, this time using rice-shochu vinegar. Feed containing this vinegar was given to mice after they were inoculated with a sarcoma and colon tumor cells. The mice that had been given the vinegar have smaller tumors than those who did not, leading researchers to suggest that the vinegar may have some anti-tumor properties.

It should be noted that most of these were studies (except for the one by Xibib and others) were performed on the cells themselves or lab animals - not on humans who were diagnosed with these types of cancers, so some caution needs to be exercised when drawing conclusions on the anti-tumor benefits of these vinegars. It appears that there are some anti-cancer benefits that vinegar does have but more studies need to be performed before any firm anti-cancer claims can be made.

Anti-diabetic Benefits

Studies also indicate that vinegar may have an anti-diabetic effect. For instance, Johnson and others studied the use of vinegar with subjects who had varying degrees of insulin sensitivity. Study participants included those who were either insulin resistant or insulin sensitive but not diabetic, as well as study subjects who were diabetic. The fasting subjects were given either a vinegar drink, which consisted of

20g of apple cider vinegar, 40g of water and 1 tsp of saccharine or a placebo. Two minutes afterward, both groups ate a small meal consisting of orange juice, a bagel and butter. Blood was drawn at fasting, and at 30 minute and 60 minute intervals after eating to determine the insulin and glucose levels. For those resistant to insulin the vinegar drink improved their sensitivity to it. Diabetics only had a slightly improved glucose level. The results showed that those who drank the vinegar had decreased changes in their glucose levels after eating. This improvement was seen in those who were insulin resistant and slightly in subjects with type 2 diabetes. Also those in the control group who received vinegar had greatly reduced changes in insulin after the meal. The results showed that those with insulin resistance who consumed vinegar had greatly decreased post-meal changes in glucose and insulin levels. The authors indicated that acetic acid has been shown to increase levels of glucose-6-phosphate as well as lower disaccharide activity in skeletal muscle. Thus, vinegar appears to work like diabetes medications like metformin and acarbose.

Anti-microbial Benefits

Studies have also shown that vinegar has anti-microbial benefits. It has been reported that using consecutive treatments of very acidic vinegar can remove warts. Similarly, diluted vinegar at 2% acetic acid with a 2 pH of 2, was useful against ear infections like granular myringitis as well as otitis media and otitis externa. Although it appears that care should be taken when using dilute vinegar for such infections. Irritation of inflamed skin as well as damage to the outer hair cells of the cochlea might occur.

Vinegar has also been reported as a screening tool in remote, poor areas like those the Amazon jungle and Zimbabwe, to detect human papilloma virus lesions in women. A 77% detection rate is seen with this method.

In contrast, according to Johnson and Gaas, the main anti-microbial benefits of vinegar come in the realm of food preparation. Placing food into vinegar is a good way to preserve it. Vinegars like apple cider vinegar or distilled white vinegar can be used for this purpose. Experts do not advice using vinegar in place of household disinfectant because the latter are more effective.

CHAPTER 3

Summary of the Health Benefits of Apple Cider and other Vinegars-with some Caveats

It must be again emphasized that more research is needed to draw any significant health conclusions to the studies provided above, as some of the study authors themselves admit. But the studies performed so far seem to indicate that there are some health benefits to using vinegar, including apple cider vinegar. Such benefits include the successful treatment of ear infections, decreasing the fluctuation in glucose and insulin levels of those who are insulin resistant, reducing the size of tumors in rats with cancer, among other potential benefits.

Although the science is still developing regarding the potential health effects of apple cider vinegar, there is no doubt that it is an established food product that has been used successfully in food preparation. For those interested in incorporating this product into their diet there are many food and drink recipes to choose from. A small sample of such recipes are below.

If you are choosing to include vinegar, including apple cider vinegar, into your diet because you are already convinced of the great health benefits that it can provide, caution should be taken. Consult with a healthcare professional like your family doctor or a registered dietician before making any drastic changes to your eating habits. Similarly, if you have a condition like diabetes, then medical advice should be sought before trying to add apple cider vinegar or other vinegars to your diet. According to Michael Danzinger, M.D., at Tufts University, diabetes lifestyle coaching program, a common condition that diabetics may have, gastroparesis in which the stomach empties itself of food slowly, may be exacerbated by the use of vinegar. Additionally, the acidity of vinegar can harm teeth enamel. So drinking it undiluted might not be a good idea. Danzinger also states that the extra acid that vinegar places into your body may harm the kidneys and bones. One study has reported low potassium levels and decreased bone density stemming from the use of apple cider vinegar. So those with osteoporosis or low potassium should take care when using it. Since it can lead to low potassium, in theory medicines like Lanoxin (digoxin) may become harmful according to alternative health expert Cathy Wong. Likewise, laxatives, insulin and diuretics like Lasix (furosemide) may become toxic. Moreover, taking in a large amount of apple cider vinegar has been shown to harm the stomach, duodenum (part of the small intestine) and liver in animals.

Therefore, again it is important to consult your doctor when adding this or any new product to your diet.

CHAPTER 4

Drink Recipes using Apple Cider Vinegar

Here is a sampling of some of the ways that apple cider and other vinegars can be used in drinks. These recipes are claiming no overt health benefit. (Note: Some of the names of the drinks are similar but the ingredients are different, making each drink unique.)

Apple Cider Vinegar Drink (6)

Ingredients:

- 2 teaspoons of apple cider vinegar
- 8 ox of water
- A packet of Splenda sugar substitute (or 1 tablespoon of natural honey)

Directions:

1. Mix the apple cider vinegar into 8 oz. of water.
2. Add a packet of Splenda or a tablespoon of honey.
3. Mix the ingredients well so that the honey or Splenda is no longer visible or barely visible in the water.
4. Drink.
5. This drink may be served warmed up, or on ice or at room temperature.

Warm Apple Cider Vinegar (20)

Ingredients:

- 1-2 cups of water
- 2 teaspoons for apple cider vinegar
- 1 tablespoon of honey

Directions:

1. Heat the water in a kettle, teapot, sauce pan.
2. Add the honey and vinegar to a mug.
3. Add the water to the mug, after the water has been heated.
4. Stir the mug contents until the honey and vinegar have dissolved.
5. Serve.

Ginger Shrub Recipe (21)(22)

Ingredients:

- 1/2 cup of finely minced ginger root
- 1 cup of apple cider vinegar
- 1/2 cup of sugar

Directions:

1. Heat the ginger and vinegar on high heat in a medium sauce pan until it starts to boil around the edges of the pan.

2. Move the liquid to a glass container and allow it to cool down.

3. Cover the glass container and allow the vinegar and ginger mixture sit at room temperature for a minimum of one day (24 hours).

4. Remove the ginger from the liquid by straining. Make certain to not press the liquid from the ginger.

5. Put the ginger and vinegar mixture in a medium saucepan and add the sugar.

6. Boil the mixture over medium heat and then reduce it to low heat, stirring occasionally, for a few minutes.

7. Let the mixture (now shrub syrup) cool and then store in the refrigerator. It can be added to juice, soda, water, or lemonade.

Basic Apple Cider Vinegar Drink (21)

Ingredients:

- 2 cups of cold water
- 1/4 cup of apple juice
- 1 tablespoons of raw apple cider vinegar
- 1 teaspoon of stevia
- Sprinkle of ground cinnamon or ground ginger

Directions:

1. Combine all the ingredients (in a pitcher) and serve cold.

Berry Shrub Recipe (21)

Ingredients:

- 1 1/2 cup of blackberries or raspberries (or a mix of both)
- 1/2 cup of apple cider vinegar
- 1/2 cup of sugar

Directions:

1. Heat the fruit and vinegar in a medium saucepan over high heat until it starts to boil around the edges of the liquid.

2. Move the mixture to a glass container and let it cool. After cooling, let it sit for a minimum of 24 hours at room temperature.

3. Strain the berries from the liquid, but do not press the liquid from the berries.

4. Place the liquid in a medium pan and add sugar. Boil the mixture over medium heat. Reduce it to a simmer, stirring occasionally, for a few minutes.

5. Cool the mixture (the shrub) and let it sit in the refrigerator.

6. When serving use 1 part shrub syrup to 10 parts of the liquid. Add the shrub syrup to water, lemonade or ginger ale.

Peach-Ginger Shrub (52)

Ingredients:

- 4 peaches
- 1/2 cup of grated fresh ginger
- 1 1/4 cup of white balsamic vinegar
- 1/2 apple cider vinegar
- 1 cup of sugar

Directions:

1. Mash the peaches in a bowl after removing the pits. Add ginger and sugar. Then stir the mixture well.

2. Cover and refrigerate for the night.

3. Press the mixture through a sieve and into a medium-size bowl.

4. Remove the peach solids.

5. Add the white balsamic and apple cider vinegar. Mix well.

6. Use a funnel to pour this vinegar and juice mixture into a bottle.

7. Seal the bottle and shake it very well.

8. Return the mixture to the refrigerator. Keep it in there for 3-5 days, shaking the bottle periodically to help dissolve the sugar.

9. After the sugar has dissolved, serve with white rum or seltzer water.

10. The drink can be kept in the refrigerator for several months.

Fresh Apple Shrub (53)

Ingredients:

- 3 medium apples (Use a variety that lots of flavor and is sweet.)
- 1 cup apple cider vinegar
- 2/3 granulated white sugar

Directions:

1. Grate the apples on a box grater.

2. Use a funnel to put the apples shreds into a wide-mouthed jar.

3. Cover the apple shreds with the vinegar and sugar. Stir the mixture together.

4. Put a watertight lid on the jar and shake well.

5. Place the jar in the back of the refrigerator for 4-5 days.

6. Do a taste test of the liquid to see if tastes right. Strain the apple pieces, removing water from the apple bits as well. You can use clean hands to do this.

7. Put the shrub in a clean container and leave in the refrigerator.

8. The shrub mixture is done but can also be allowed to sit for awhile, as the flavors mature over time.

9. Use the apple shrub for vinaigrettes or marinades. It can also be used in drinks by mixing it with seltzer water or cocktails.

Apple Cider Vinegar Brew (54)

Ingredients:

- 1/2 cup of water
- 1/4 cup of unfiltered apple cider vinegar
- 1 tsp of cayenne pepper
- 1 tbsp honey
- 1 wedge lemon

Directions:

1. Boil the water.

2. Mix the hot water and the apple cider vinegar and in a small mug or glass.

3. Add cayenne pepper and honey.

4. Mix well.

5. Put a wedge of lemon at the top and drink.

Raspberry Shrub (55)

Ingredients:

- 24-30 organic fresh or frozen raspberries
- Optional, two stalks of lemongrass
- 25 ounces (or 750 milliliters) of coconut vinegar (5% acidity)
- 1/2 cup of sugar, more to taste

Directions:

1. Put the lemongrass (optional), raspberries and vinegar in a non-reactive container like quality glass or plastic.

2. Seal the container and let it sit for 3-5 days on the counter at room temperature. Stir the mixture once or twice each day. The berries will be broken down in a 1 or 2.

3. Transfer the berries and vinegar to a small pan and stir in the 1/2 cup of sugar.

4. Bring the berries, vinegar and sugar mixture to a boil over med-high heat and then lower the heat to a simmer. Very gently simmer for 1 hour.

5. Strain 1 to 2 teaspoons of the mixture into a glass and allow to cool. Add seltzer water and taste. Add sugar if needed and then remove from heat and allow it to cool down for 15-20 minutes.

6. Strain the mixture over a mesh strainer placed over a bowl. Make sure to press as much juice out of the fruit pulp as possible.

7. Strain liquid through a mesh strainer lined with several layers of cheese cloth into a large container, at least the size of a quart.

8. Move mixture to a bottle. Cool the mixture to room temperature, then seal and store it in the refrigerator.

9. Use for whatever food or drink you desire.

New York Shrub (56)

Ingredients:

- 1/2 cup of balsamic vinegar
- 1 1/2 house cup of Rittenhouse Rye
- 3/4 cup of fresh lemon juice
- 1/2 cup of simple syrup

Directions:

1. For the simple syrup, pour 1 cup of water and 1 cup of sugar in a saucepan. Heat over medium heat, while stirring until the sugar is dissolved. Cool prior to use.

2. Pour balsamic vinegar into a sauce pan and boil.

3. Let it simmer until it reduces to half its volume. This will take about 10 minutes.

4. Let it cool to room temperature.

5. To make the cocktail, pour the rye, simple syrup, lemon and 1 barspoon (1 teaspoon) of the vinegar reduction into a cocktail shaker. Fill with ice and shake until it is well chilled. This will take about 15 seconds.

6. Pour into an ice-filled rocks glass.

CHAPTER 5

Food Recipes using Apple Cider Vinegar

Here are some food recipes that use apple cider vinegar or other types of vinegar as an ingredient. Again no overt health claims are being promoted by including these recipes.

Grilled Apple Cider Vinegar Chicken(8)

Ingredients: *(For chicken and brine)*

- 1/3 cup of firmly packed light brown sugar
- 3/4 cup of Kosher salt
- 6-8 pieces from a 4-5 pound chicken
- Black pepper, freshly ground

Ingredients: *(basting liquid)*

1. 1/2 cup of apple cider vinegar
2. 2 tablespoons of Worcestershire sauce
3. 1/4 cup of canola oil, plus more for the grill grate
4. 1 tablespoon of hot sauce, or to taste

Directions:

For the chicken and the brine:

1. Add brown sugar, salt and 1 gallon of cold water to a large plastic container and stir until the solids are dissolved.

2. Prepare a charcoal barbeque, making certain that the charcoals have a thin grey film on them before the chicken is cooked on the barbeque. This film should be available after about 20-30 minutes. (For gas grills, turn the grill on to hot, and close the lid for 10-15 minutes.)

For the basting liquid:

1. Mix together the apple cider vinegar, Worcestershire sauce, hot sauce, oil and 1/2 cup of water using a whisk. Set this mixture aside.

2. Drain the chicken, pat dry and shake black pepper over it.

3. Add some oil to the grill grate.

4. Place the chicken pieces on the grill grate, leaving some space between the pieces. Baste the chicken pieces with the basting liquid.

5. Let the chicken stay on the grill until seared (or for about 1-2 minutes.)

6. Transfer the chicken to a cooler part of the grill and let cook until the juices in the chicken run clear when the pieces are pierced with a fork. This should be about 18-20 minutes.

7. Serve!

Garden Salad with Apple Cider Viniagrette(16)

Ingredients:

- 2 cups apple cider
- 1/4 apple cider vinegar
- 1/4 cup honey
- 1 cinnamon stick
- 2 cups grapeseed oil
- 6 cups of loosely packed mixed greens like romaine, radicchio, and red and green lettuce
- Freshly ground black pepper
- Salt
- 2 cup of assorted berries (raspberries, blackberries, blueberries, etc.)
- Granny Smith apples, cored and sliced
- 1 1/2 cups of crumbled blue cheese

Directions:

1. In a jar or bowl with a tight lid combine the apple cider vinegar, honey, apple cider, oil, cinnamon, pepper and salt. In a large bowl place the greens, blue cheese, apples and berries together. Toss them and cover the salad with the dressing so that there is enough to coat everything. Add pepper and salt. Serve.

(Apple) Cider Vinegar-Spiked Baby Spinach (17)

Ingredients:

- 1 16 oz. container of baby spinach leaves
- 2 tablespoons of apple cider vinegar
- 1 tablespoon of water
- 1/8 teaspoon of Kosher salt
- 1/4 teaspoon of crush red pepper flakes

Directions:

1. Place spinach in a large bowl.
2. Cover the bowl with plastic wrap.
3. Microwaves the leaves on high until the spinach wilts.
4. Drain
5. Toss with red pepper flakes, vinegar, and salt.

Green Beans with a Cider Glaze(19)

Ingredients:

- 1 pound of fresh green beans
- 2 tablespoons of butter
- 1 medium red onion (sliced lengthwise)
- 3/4 cup of apple cider
- 3 tablespoons of apple cider vinegar
- 1 teaspoon of salt
- 1/2 teaspoon of freshly ground chili pepper
- 2 teaspoons of Dijon mustard

Directions:

1. Boil the beans until they are crispy and tender. This should be for about 5 minutes. Drain.

2. Cook the onions and butter in a skillet over medium heat for 2 minutes.

3. Add apple cider vinegar and apple cider to the skillet with the onions and butter. Cook until the liquid has almost disappeared. It should take about 7 minutes.

4. Stir in the salt, chili pepper, and mustard. Add the beans to the skillet and stir until the mixture is heated through.

Strawberries with Balsamic Vinegar (18)

Ingredients:

- 4 cups of strawberries, cut in half
- 1 tablespoon of sugar
- 1 tablespoon of balsamic vinegar

Directions:

1. Combine the ingredients in a bowl, making certain to toss very well.

2. Let the mixture sit for 30 minutes.

3. Toss again before serving.

~ ❖ ~

Apple Cider and Vinegar Mop Sauce (57)

Ingredients:

- 1 tbsp butter
- 1/2 cup diced onions (about 1/2 small onion)
- 1 tbsp chopped garlic
- 1 tbsp paprika

- 1 teaspoon dried mustard powder
- 1 bay leaf
- 2 cups of apple cider
- 1 1/2 cup of ketchup
- 1 crushed chipotle in adobo sauce
- 1/2 cup of apple cider vinegar

Directions:

1. Melt the butter over a medium heat.

2. Add onion and garlic. Cook them for about 4 minutes, stirring the mixture until the onions are almost clear.

3. Add the paprika, mustard seed and bay leaf.

4. Cook this until it is aromatic. This should take about 30 seconds.

5. Add the cider, chipotle and ketchup. Bring them to a simmer and cook until the sauce thickens a little. This should take about 15 minutes.

6. Add the cider vinegar and cook for another 5 minutes. The mop sauce is done. It should be thin in consistency and tart in flavor.

7. Continue to cook the sauce for another 20-30 minutes to create the barbeque sauce. Season to taste.

Smoky Chicken and Cider (58)

Ingredients:

- Extra virgin olive oil
- 8 oz. good-quality sliced smokey bacon
- 8-10 pieces of bone-in chicken legs, thighs and breast meat
- Kosher salt and freshly ground black pepper
- 2 onions peeled and cut into wedges with the root end attached
- 4 carrots, peeled and sliced on an angle 1/2 inches thick
- 2 tablespoons of fresh, chopped thyme
- 2-3 large fresh bay leaves
- 3 tbsp of all-purpose flour
- 2 cups of cloudy apple cider
- About 1/3 cup of dark maple syrup
- 1/4 cup of apple cider vinegar
- 1 to 2 cups of chicken stock
- 1 pound of Yukon gold potatoes, quarters
- 2 golden delicious apples, quarters, sliced and cored

Directions:

1. Heat a drizzle of extra-virgin olive oil in a large Dutch oven. Use medium heat. Add bacon and remove from the oven, after it browns.

2. Season pieces of chicken with salt and pepper liberally.

3. Brown the chicken meat on both sides in two batches.

4. Remove them from the pan onto a plate.

5. Add the thyme, onions, bay leaves, carrots, to the Dutch oven and season with pepper and salt.

6. Cover the pan. Cook the vegetables for 5 to 6 minutes, until they are tender. Stir occasionally.

7. Add the flour and stir 1-2 minutes, then add the apple cider, vinegar, syrup, 1 cup chicken stock.

8. Add the potatoes and apples and add the bacon on top.

9. Place the chicken in the pan and add chicken stock until the liquid goes to the edge, but do not cover the chicken.

10. Cover the pan, lower the heat and cook the chicken through. This should take about 15 minutes.

11. Cool and refrigerate to eat later.

12. Reheat in an oven that is preheated to 325 degrees F or on the stove over medium heat covered until it is completely warmed up.

13. Serve immediately.

14. Remove the cooked chicken to a shallow bowls or a serving platter. Stir to thicken and combine the vegetables and sauce. Spoon this over and around the chicken.

Vinegar French Fries (59)

Ingredients:

- Four Russet potatoes cut into 1/4 inch strips
- 4 tablespoons of distilled white vinegar
- Vegetable oil for frying
- Kosher salt

Directions:

1. Soak the potatoes in cold water so that it covers the potatoes.

2. Stir in 2 tablespoons of vinegar. Put the potatoes in the refrigerator for 1 to 4 hours.

3. Pour 3 inches of vgetable oil in to a large Dutch oven. Heat the oil until it reaches 325 degrees F.

4. Strain potatoes from the water. Dry them completely.

5. Fry the potatoes in the hot oil. Do not fry them all at once, but in batches. Remove the first batch of cooked potatoes from the oil with a slotted spoon or spider. Using this sort of cooking utensil prevents the potatoes from sticking to each other. The potatoes should be removed when they are light brown. The frying at this stage should take about 4 minutes.

6. Put the fries on a cooking rack. Increase the temperature of the oil to 375 degrees F.

7. Fry the potatoes a second time in order to get them to be golden brown. This should take about 2-3 minutes.

8. Toss the 2 tbsp of vinegar on the fries. Season with salt.

9. Enjoy.

~ ❖ ~

Peanut Butter Chicken Wings, Rice Noodle Salad with Peanut Crunch and Rice Wine Vinegar Dressing (60)

Ingredients:

(Peanut Butter Chicken Wing Marinade)

- cups of smooth natural peanut butter
- 1/2 cup of brown sugar
- 8 cloves of garlic, minced
- Zest of 1 lime
- 1 teaspoon of cayenne pepper
- 1/2 teaspoon of freshly ground black pepper
- 1 cup of soy sauce
- 1/2 cup of water
- Juice of two limes

(Peanut Butter Chicken Wings)

- 24 chicken wings
- Peanut butter chicken wing marinade

(Peanut Crunch)

- Peanut oil, for frying
- 2 red finger chilies, haled, seeded and sliced
- 2 shallots, halved, peeled and sliced
- 5 tbsp of cornstarch
- Salt
- 1 cup of chopped toasted peanuts

(Rice Wine Vinegar Salad Dressing)

- 1 cup of seasoned rice wine vinegar
- 1 clove of garlic minced
- 1 tsp of sesame oil
- Zest of 1 lime
- Salt

(Rice Noodle Salad)

- 1 (8 oz./227g) package of vermicelli rice noodles cooked according the package directions
- 1 cucumber, peeled and seeded
- 1/2 bunch of green onions, sliced on a thin bias
- 1/2 bunch of fresh cilantro, leaves picked
- Peanut butter chicken wings
- Rice wine vinegar dressing
- Peanut butter crunch
- 2 cups of bean sprouts
- 1 carrot, peeled and julienned.

Directions:

(For the peanut butter chicken wing marinade)

1. Put peanut butter, brown sugar, lime zest, garlic, black pepper, cayenne pepper, water, soy sauce, and lime juice in a large bowl.

(For the peanut butter chicken wings)

1. Score the chicken wings to allow the marinade to penetrate the meat.

2. Put the chicken wings in the peanut butter marinade.

3. Massage the marinade on the wings. Place the wings in the refrigerator for 30 minutes to a maximum of 24 hours.

4. Preheat the oven to 350 degrees F.

5. Place parchment paper on a large baking tray.

6. Place the wings on a tray. Bake in the oven, turning them over half way through the cooking time. Cook until the wings are crisp and golden brown. This should take about 30-45 minutes.

(For the Peanut Butter Crunch)

1. Fill a large heavy-bottomed pot 1/3 full of oil.

2. Check the temperature using a deep-fry thermometer. Heat the oils to 350 degrees F.

3. Line a baking sheet with a paper towel.

4. Place the chilies in a bowl.

5. Coat liberally with 2 tablespoon of cornstarch. Fry until golden brown.

6. Remove from the oil and place on a paper-lined baking tray and season with salt. Lay to the side.

7. Place the shallots and chilies on a cutting board. Finely chop them.

8. Mix the chopped chilies, shallots and peanuts in a bowl and set aside.

(For Rice Wine Vinegar Dressing)

1. Put the seasoned rice wine vinegar, garlic, sesame oil, salt and lime vest in a bowl.

2. Stir and set aside.

(To assemble)

1. Position the rice noodles in the center of the plate. Dress with 1/2 of the rice wine vinegar dressing.

2. Add the peanut crunch over the noodles. Put the bean sprouts over the rice noodles.

3. Place the carrots around the outside of the bean sprouts and rice noodles.

4. Scatter the green onions and cucumber over the carrots then place the remaining rice wine vinegar over them.

5. Put the peanut butter chicken wings over the rice noodles and garnish with the cilantro.

Baked Kale Chips with Apple Cider Vinegar (61)

Ingredients:

- 1 bunch kale, rinsed, steamed and thoroughly dried
- 1/4 cup of olive oil
- Sea salt
- Sufficient amount of apple cider vinegar

Directions:

(Kale Chips)

1. Preheat an oven to 350 degrees F. Add oil and kale to a plastic bag.

2. Seal the bag and distribute the oil as evenly as possible on the kale.

3. Spread the kale onto a baking sheet evenly.

4. Cook until crispy (for about 10-15 minutes).

5. Remove from the oven.

6. Sprinkle with sea salt and vinegar

7. Enjoy.

CHAPTER 6

Getting Reliable Information about Natural Health Remedies, Including the Apple Cider Vinegar Weight Loss "Secret"

From the Atkins Diet to the South Beach Diet, there have been many health food and diet trends that have been marketed over the passed several decades. This is no surprise. Obesity is a major health problem in the US, as it is throughout the world, in developed and developing countries. So creating quick ways to lose weight can be an understandable way to deal with a difficult and widespread health issue. Certainly, being overweight or obese is not about having a few extra pounds. It can lead to a large number of serious health problems including type 2 diabetes, respiratory problems such as sleep apnea, various cancers (like those of the breast, colon and endometrium), cardiovascular problems like heart attacks, strokes, and hypertension, destruction of joint cartilage, as well as some mental health problems. (It has been observed that there is a link between obesity and depression, as well as potentially other mental health problems.)

Thus the issue of excessive weight gain should be dealt with, but in a thoughtful and reasonable manner. Therefore, it should be said that there is no apple cider vinegar weight loss "secret." Simply following the most recent health trend is not always a good idea and it may even be harmful. For example, utilizing apple cider vinegar to help lose weight may be effective for some. But researchers have noted that vinegar is very acidic. Therefore, it may harm the stomach of some people, therefore, making its use for weight loss problematic. Also undiluted vinegar can harm one's teeth by eroding the enamel. Maintaining a healthy weight is important for good heath but should not come at the expense of harming a specific part of your body. Therefore, gaining the right information on how to safely lose weight is important for meaningful weight loss.

It is an established fact that to lose weight you have to eat a balanced diet, (consuming the daily recommended amount of calories to lose weight), get regular exercise and enough sleep daily. These are general guidelines which do not take into account the specific issues that a person who is trying to lose weight might face, further highlighting the fact that people should be careful about following healthcare trends. Each person's weight loss plan should be tailored to himself or herself. For example, even with getting enough sleep, eating a balanced diet and getting regular exercise, some people may still have trouble losing weight due to a chemical imbalance within their bodies like an underactive thyroid. Difficulties losing weight may even stem from some type of emotional problem, or a combination of factors.

Additionally, there is the issue of details. Eating a balanced diet, getting regular exercise and sleeping enough sound simple, but what exactly does it mean, especially since the diet, exercise and sleep needs of a person may change based on their age, health conditions they may be dealing with or other factors. Eating a balanced diet can mean different things to different people. For instance, the food preferences and needs of an adult age 75 may be different from an adult aged 25. The sleep needs may differ as well since typically the older you get, the less sleep you need. Additionally, the type of physical activity that you may do as a young person may differ from what you can do as an older adult. Therefore, a weight loss plan needs to take into account your age, gender (women typically require less calories than men), your level of fitness, what sort of health conditions you may have, among other things.

So when trying to lose weight and live a healthier lifestyle, how can you get the right information? The most obvious answer is a good place to start: talk to your doctor. Depending on your doctor's level of expertise in the matter and your specific needs, she or he may recommend you to a specialist like a nutritionist, a registered dietician, an endocrinologist or even a psychologist. There are many reasons why a person gains weight and therefore, there can be a myriad of ways in which to deal with reducing your weight.

Along with talking to your doctor about weight loss, you may want to consult other resources, especially if you are interested in doing it without taking medications. Reliable resources on natural health include the website for the National Center for Complementary and Integrative Medicine which discusses what complementary or alternative medicine is and the types of therapies that have been studied as well as supplements. Much of the information is directed at a lay audience. For health professionals, there are copies of abstracts with more details on the research scientists have conducted. For natural and alternative medicines, not a lot of research has been done, but some studies that have been published. Additionally, the NIH website also carries information on dietary supplements on its Office of Dietary Supplements webpages and information about herbal medicine and other alternative treatments is located on the Medline Plus webpages. Another helpful resource for alternative medicine is drugs.com. The website lists various medications, including vitamins, their uses, side effects and possible interactions with other medications or foods, and even recipes for healthy eating. There are also stores which specifically sell natural therapies which stem from health traditions outside the US. For instance, in Chicago, Illinois the store Merz Apothocary carries various health and beauty products from around the world, such as comfrey root, which is traditional in Chinese medicine. The root has been studied and shown to help those with pain, including back pain. Other trusted sources of information about natural remedies or health supplements include the websites WebMD and Medicinenet.

REFERENCES:

1. Mermel, V. L. (2004). Old paths new Directions: the use of functional foods in the treatment of obesity. *Trends in Food Science & Technology*, 15(11), 532-540. Abstract. Retrieved from http://www.sciencedirect.com/science/article/pii/S0924224404001414

2. Budak, N. H., Aykin, E. Seydim, A.C., Greene, A.K., & Guzel-Seydim, Z. B., (2014) Functional Properties of Vinegar. *Journal of Food Science*, 79(5), 757-764. DOI: 10.1111/1750-3841.12434

3. Nelson, J. K. (2012, June 9) I've heard the term "functional foods," but I don't know what it means. Can you explain? Retrieved from http://www.mayoclinic.org/healthy-living/nutrition-and-healthy-eating/expert-answers/functional-foods/faq-20057816

4. Manning, J. (2014, October 1) Apple Cider Vinegar and Health. Retrieved from http://www.webmd.com/diet/features/apple-cider-vinegar-and-health

5. White, D.A. (2013, June 27) Apple Cider Vinegar: Worth the Hype? Retrieved from http://blog.foodnetwork.com/healthyeats/2013/06/27/apple-cider-vinegar-worth-the-hype/

6. Cooks, S. (2010, March 10) Apple Cider Vinegar Cocktail. Retrieved from http://www.food.com/recipe/apple-cider-vinegar-cocktail-418526

7. Willis, V. Grilled Apple Cider Vinegar Chicken. Retrieved from http://www.foodnetwork.com/recipes/grilled-apple-cider-vinegar-chicken.html

8. Szwarc, S. (2008, April 3) Houston...we have a problem-Apple cider vinegar remedies. Retrieved from http://junkfoodscience.blogspot.com/search?q=apple+cider+vinegar

9. Johnston, C.S. & Gaas, C.A. (2006) Vinegar: Medicinal Uses and Antiglycemic Effect. *Medscape General Medicine*. 81(2), 61 Retrieved from http://www.ncbi.nlm.nih.gov/pmc/articles/PMC1785201/

10. The University of Sydney. (2014) About Glycemic Index. Retrieved from http://www.glycemicindex.com/about.php

11. Sharon, NA. (2013, May 17) Homemade Apple Cider Vinegar. Retrieved from http://www.food.com/recipe/homemade-apple-cider-vinegar-500431

12. Joybilee Farm. (2012) How to make apple cider vinegar at home using apple cider. Retrieved from http://joybileefarm.com/make-apple-cider-vinegar/

13. How Products are Made: Vinegar. Retrieved on February 9, 2015 from http://www.madehow.com/Volume-7/Vinegar.html

14. Formaggio Kitchen. Balsamic Vinegar. Retrieved February, 9, 2015 from http://www.formaggiokitchen.com/education/balsamic_vinegar

15. McCargo, A. Glazed Salmon with Braised Fennel. Retrieved February 9, 2015 from http://www.foodnetwork.com/videos/glazed-salmon-with-fennel-0138009.html

16. Irvine, R. Garden Salad with Apple Cider Vinaigrette. Retrieved February 9, 2015 from http://www.foodnetwork.com/recipes/robert-irvine/garden-salad-with-apple-cider-vinaigrette-recipe.html

17. Hobbs, K. (2014, May) Cider Vinegar-Spiked Steamed Baby Spinach. Retrieved from http://www.myrecipes.com/recipe/spiked-steamed-baby-spinach

18. Day, S. (1995, May) Strawberries with Balsamic Vinegar. Retrieved from http://www.myrecipes.com/recipe/strawberries-with-balsamic-vinegar

19. Recipeland. (2008, October 3, updated February 9, 2015) Green Beans With Cider Glaze (Thanksgiving). Retrieved from http://recipeland.com/recipe/v/green-beans-cider-glaze-thanksg-47911

20. Owlett, NA. My Apple Cider Vinegar Drink. Retrieved February 9, 2015 from http://recipes.sparkpeople.com/recipe-detail.asp?recipe=646490

21. Woods, C. Don't Be Grossed Out! Try These Apple Cider Vinegar Drink Recipes. Retrieved February 9, 2015 http://www.vegan-nutritionista.com/apple-cider-vinegar-drink.html

22. Han, E. How to Make a Fruit Shrub Syrup. Retrieved from http://www.thekitchn.com/how-to-make-a-shrub-syrup-174072

23. Hondo, T., Kishi, M., Fushimim, T., Ugajin, S. KagaT. (2009) Vinegar intake reduces body weight, body fat mass, and serum triglyceride levels in obese Japanese subjects. *Bioscience, Biochemistry and Biotechnology*, 73(8), 1837-43. Abstract. Retrieved from http://www.ncbi.nlm.nih.gov/pubmed/?term=PMID%3A+19661687

24. Lab Tests Online. (2011, September 20) ACE. Retrieved from http://labtestsonline.org/understanding/analytes/ace/tab/test

25. Honcho, S., A. Sugiyama, Takahara, A., Satoh, Y., Nakamura, Y., Hashimoto, K. (2005) A red wine vinegar beverage can inhibit the renin-angiotensin system: experimental evidence in vivo. *Biological & Pharmaceutical Bulletin*. 28(7) 1208-1210. Retrieved from http://ci.nii.ac.jp/els/10016665252.pdf?id=ART0004208360&type=pdf&lang=en&host=cinii&order_no=&ppv_type=0&lang_sw=&no=1423060585&cp=

26. Sugiyama, K., Sakakibara, R., Tachimoto, H., Kishi, M., Kaga, T., Tabata, I., (2010) Effects of Acetic Acid Bacteria Supplementation On Muscle Damage After Moderate-Intensity Exercise. *Japanese Society of Anti-Aging Medicine*, 7(1), 1-6. Retrieved from http://www.anti-aging.gr.jp/english/pdf/2010/ms6-17_7-1.pdf

27. Medical News Today (2014, September 2) What is inflammation? What causes inflammation? Retrieved from http://www.medicalnewstoday.com/articles/248423.php

28. Medical Health Tests (2012, March 27) Comprehensive Information on Creatine Kinase (CK). Medical Health Tests. Retrieved from http://www.medicalhealthtests.com/creatine-kinase.html

29. Kenton College (2010) Acetobacter. Retrieved from http://microbewiki.kenyon.edu/index.php/Acetobacter

30. Fukami, H., Kobayaski, S., Tachimoto, H., Kishi, M., Kaga, T., Waki, H., ...Tanaka, Y., (2010) Effect of Continuous Ingestion of Acetic Acid Bacteria on Memory Retention and the Synaptic Function in Aged Rats. *Bioscience, Biotechnology and Biochemisty*. 74(7)1498-1500. Retrieved from http://www.tandfonline.com/doi/pdf/10.1271/bbb.100164

31. The Editors of Encyclopedia Britannica. Sphingolipid. (2015) Encyclopædia Britannica. Retrieved from http://www.britannica.com/EBchecked/topic/559707/sphingolipid

32. Mimura, A., Suzuki, Y., Toshima, Y., Yazaki, S., Ohtsuki, T., Ui, S., Hyodoh, F., (2004). Induction of apoptosis in human leukemia cells by naturally fermented sugar cane vinegar (kibizu) of Amami Ohshima Island. *Biofactors*. 22(1-4), 93-97. Abstract. Retrieved from http://www.readcube.com/articles/10.1002%2Fbiof.5520220118?r3_referer=wol&tracking_action=previe w_click&show_checkout=1

33. Nanda, K., Miyoshi, N., Nakamura, Y., Shimoji, Y., Tamura, Y., Nishikawa, Y., . . . Tanaka, T. (2004) Extract of vinegar "Kurosu" from unpolished rice inhibits the proliferation of human cancer cells. *Journal of Experimental Clinical Cancer Research* 23(1), 69-75, Abstract. Retrieved from http://www.ncbi.nlm.nih.gov/pubmed/15149153

34. Johnston, C.S., Kim, C.M., & Buller, A.J., (2004) Vinegar Improves Insulin Sensitivity to a High-Carbohydrate Meal in Subjects with Insulin Resistance or Type 2 Diabetes, *Diabetes Care* 27(1), 281-282. Retrieved from http://care.diabetesjournals.org/content/27/1/281.long

35. Tran, M. (2014, January 3) Obesity soars to "alarming" levels in developing countries. Retrieved from http://www.theguardian.com/global-development/2014/jan/03/obesity-soars-alarming-levels-developing-countries

36. Centers for Disease Control and Prevention (2011, May 2011) Obesity: Halting the Epidemic by Making Health Easier At a Glance 2011. Retrieved from http://www.cdc.gov/chronicdisease/resources/publications/AAG/obesity.htm

37. Mayo Clinic Staff. (2012, December 1) Hypothyroidism (underactive thyroid). Retrieved from http://www.mayoclinic.org/diseases-conditions/hypothyroidism/basics/definition/con-20021179

38. National Institutes of Health. Teacher's Guide: Information about Sleep. Retrieved from http://www.science.education.nih.gov/supplements/nih3/sleep/guide/info-sleep.htm

39. National Center for Complementary and Integrative Health. PubMed Dietary Supplement Subset. Retrieved February 9, 2015 from http://ods.od.nih.gov/Research/PubMed_Dietary_Supplement_Subset.aspx

40. Mayo Foundation for Medical Education and Research. (2009) Berries marinated in balsamic vinegar. Retrieved from http://www.drugs.com/mcr/berries-marinated-in-balsamic-vinegar

41. Merz Apothocary. (2015) In the Press. Retrieved from http://www.smallflower.com/press/index.cfm

42. Herman, Marilyn. (2014) Vinegar for Pickling. Retrieved from http://www.extension.umn.edu/food/food-safety/preserving/pickling/vinegar-for-pickling/

43. Ho, A. (2010, October 24) Q&A: Kombucha SCOBYs vs. Mothers of Vinegar (MOVs). Retrieved from http://www.kombuchafuel.com/2010/10/kombucha-scobys-vs-mothers-of-vinegar.html

44. NA, Jessica. Emilia-Romagna. Retrieved February 9, 2014 from http://www.italylogue.com/emilia-romagna

45. Webber, C. & Shrefler, J., (2006) Vinegar as a burn-down herbicide. Acetic acid concentrations, application volumes, and adjuvants. *Oklahoma Agriculture Experiment Station Departmental Publication.* MP-162, 29-30 Retrieved from http://ars.usda.gov/research/publications/publications.htm?seq_no_115=195808

46. Jung, H.H., Cho, S.D., Yoo, C.K., Lim, H.H., Chae, S.W., (2002) Vinegar treatment in the management of granular myringitis. *Journal of Laryngology and Otology*, 116(3), 176-180. Retrieved from http://www.ncbi.nlm.nih.gov/pubmed/11893257/

47. Xibin, S., Meilan, H., Moller, H., Evans, H.S., Dixin, D., Wenjie, D., Jianbang, L., (2003) Risk Factors for Oesophageal Cancer in Linzhou, China: A Case Control Study. *Asian Pacific Journal of Cancer Prevention* 4 119-124 http://www.apocpcontrol.org/paper_file/issue_abs/Volume4_No2/Sun%20Xibin.pdf

48. Cancer Treatment Centers of America. Adenocarcinoma. Retrieved February 9, 2015 from http://www.cancercenter.com/terms/adenocarcinoma/

49. Shimoji, Y., Kohno, H., Nanda, K., Nishikawa, Y., Ohigashi, H., Tanaka, T., (2004). Extract of Kurosu, a vinegar from unpolished rice, inhibits azoxymethane-induced colon carcinogenesis in male F344 rats. *Nutrition and Cancer*, 49(2) 170-173. Retrieved from http://www.ncbi.nlm.nih.gov/pubmed/15489210

50. Seki, T., Morimura, S., Shigematsu, T., Maeda, H., Kida, K., (2004). Anti-tumor activity of rice-shochu post-distillation slurry and vinegar produced from the post-distillation slurry via oral administration in a mouse model. *Biofactors* 22(1-4) 103-105, Retrieved from http://www.ncbi.nlm.nih.gov/pubmed/15630262

51. Wong, C. (2015, January 10) Apple Cider Vinegar: What Should I know About It? Retrieved from http://altmedicine.about.com/od/applecidervinegardiet/a/applecidervineg.htm

52. Serious Eats. Peach-Ginger Shrub. Retrieved February 9, 2015 from http://www.yummly.com/recipe/Peach-ginger-shrub-302349?columns=3&position=10%2F67

53. McClellan, M., (2012, October 9) Fresh Apple Shrub. Retrieved from http://www.yummly.com/recipe/external/Fresh-apple-shrub-332425

54. Fuhr, L., (2015, January 1) Soothe That Sinus Pain: Apple Cider Vinegar Brew. Retrieved from http://www.yummly.com/recipe/external/Apple-Cider-Vinegar-Brew-900117

55. Food 52, (2011, June 6) Raspberry Shrub (aka Drinking Vinegar). Retrieved from http://www.yummly.com/recipe/external/Raspberry-shrub-_aka-drinking-vinegar_-326352

56. Hoffman, M. (2012, December 12) New York Shrub. Retrieved from http://www.yummly.com/recipe/external/New-york-shrub-304915

57. Camillo, V., Apple Cider BBQ Mop and Sauce. Retrieved February 09, 2015 from http://www.cookingchanneltv.com/recipes/apple-cider-bbq-mop-and-sauce.html

58. Ray, R., Smoky Chicken and Cider. Retrieved February, 9, 2015 from http://www.cookingchanneltv.com/recipes/rachael-ray/smoky-chicken-and-cider.html

59. Loo, S., Vinegar French Fries. Retrieved February 9, 2015 from http://www.cookingchanneltv.com/recipes/vinegar-french-fries.html

60. Mooking, R., Peanut Butter Chicken Wings, Rice Noodle Salad with Peanut Crunch and Rice Wine Vinegar Dressing. Retrieved February 9, 2015 from http://www.cookingchanneltv.com/recipes/roger-mooking/peanut-butter-chicken-wings-rice-noodle-salad-with-peanut-crunch-and-rice-wine-vinegar-dressing.html

61. Giosia, N. Baked Kale Chips with Cider Vinegar. Retrieved February 9, 2015 from http://www.cookingchanneltv.com/recipes/nadia-g/baked-kale-chips-with-cider-vinegar.html

62. Mercola, J.M., (2009, June 2) What Research Really Says About Apple Cider Vinegar. http://articles.mercola.com/sites/articles/archive/2009/06/02/apple-cider-vinegar-hype.aspx

CONCLUSION

This book was written with the intention of briefly educating the reader on some of the latest research and understanding related to apple cider vinegar and other vinegars, regarding weight loss and health. It is hoped that rather than simply jumping on the "band-wagon" of yet another healthcare trend, the reader decides to get more information before adding apple cider vinegar or anything else new to their diet. As the old saying goes, there's nothing more important than your health. So rather than letting random claims about a food guide your decision-making process, seek to make good health choices for yourself by getting the right information from a variety of sources in order to make an informed decision.

To hear about Jessica's new books first (and to be notified when there are free promotions), sign up to her New Release Mailing List.

Finally, if you enjoyed this book, please take the time to share your thoughts and post a review on Amazon. It'd be greatly appreciated!

Pear Chicken Curry

SERVES 6

Ingredients:

- 2 ripe pears, divided

- 1 tablespoon vegetable oil

- 1 cup onion, diced

- 1 tablespoon curry powder

- 1 teaspoon minced garlic

- 1 teaspoon salt

- 3/4 teaspoon ground ginger

- 3/4 teaspoon ground cinnamon

- 1/4 teaspoon ground black pepper

- 3 chicken breasts, halved, boneless, skinless, cut into 1 inch cubes

- 1 can light coconut milk

- 1/3 cup raisins

Preparation:

Peel and core 1 pear. Puree and set aside.

Heat oil in a frying pan over medium heat. Add onion, curry powder, garlic, salt, ginger, cinnamon, and pepper. Sauté for 5 minutes, stirring occasionally or until onions are transparent.

Add chicken and continue to sauté 5 minutes, stirring occasionally or until browned. Add pureed pear, coconut milk, and raisins. Simmer for 5 minutes. Core and cut remaining pear into 1/2 inch cubes and add to curry. Simmer for 5 minutes. Serve.

Nutrition Information:

272 calories, 10 g total fat, 5 g saturated fat, 20 g carbohydrate, 24 g protein, 3.5 g fiber, 452 mg sodium, 383 mg potassium, 31 mg magnesium, 35 mg calcium

MORE BOOKS ON FOOD, HEALTH AND WELLNESS

Click here to check out the rest of Jessica's books on Amazon.

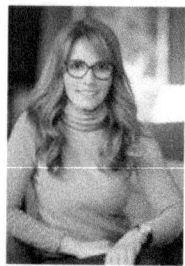

Below you'll find some of my other popular books that are popular on Amazon and Kindle as well. Simply click on the links below to check them out. Alternatively, you can visit my author page on Amazon to see other work done by me.

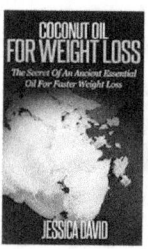 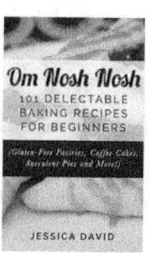 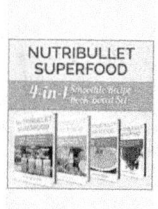 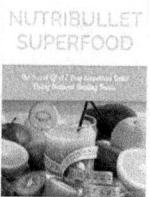 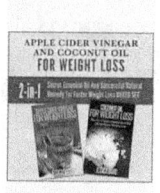

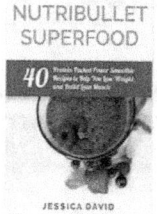 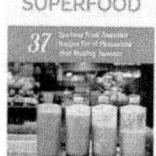 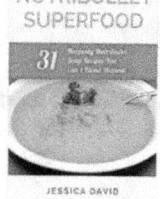 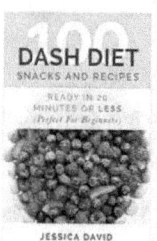 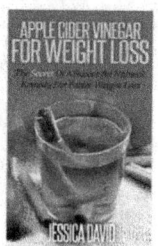

Nutribullet Superfood: 31 Heavenly Nutribullet Soup Recipes You Can't Blend Without

Nutribullet Superfood: The Secret Of A 7 Day Smoothies Detox Using Natural Healing Foods

Nutribullet Superfood: 40 Protein Packed Power Smoothie Recipes To Help You Lose Weight And Build Lean Muscle (Includes: Bonus Protein Add-Ins Guide)

Nutribullet Superfood: 37 Luscious Fruit Smoothie Recipes For A Pleasurable And Healthy Summer

Nutribullet Superfood: 4-in-1 Smoothie Recipe Book Boxed Set

Dash Diet: 100 Dash Diet Snacks And Recipes: Ready In 20 Minutes Or Less (Perfect For Beginners)

Om Nosh Nosh: 101 Delectable Baking Recipes For Beginners (Gluten-Free Pastries, Coffee Cakes, Succulent Pies And More!)

Apple Cider Vinegar For Weight Loss: The Secret Of A Successful Natural Remedy For Faster Weight Loss

Coconut Oil For Weight Loss: The Secret Of An Ancient Essential Oil For Faster Weight Loss

Apple Cider Vinegar and Coconut Oil for Weight Loss: 2-in-1 Secret Essential Oil And Successful Natural Remedy For Faster Weight Loss Boxed Set

Baby Powder: 17 Impressive Uses for Baby Powder You've Never Considered

If the links do not work, for whatever reason, you can simply search for these titles on the Amazon website to find them.

COCONUT OIL
FOR WEIGHT LOSS

The Secret Of An Ancient Essential
Oil For Faster Weight Loss

JESSICA DAVID

Book 2: Coconut Oil For Weight Loss

The Secret Of An Ancient Essential Oil
For Faster Weight Loss

Jessica David

COPYRIGHT

Copyright © 2015

DISCLAIMER

Your Free Gift

As a special Thank You for downloading this book I have put together an exclusive report on "Superfoods For Weight Loss".

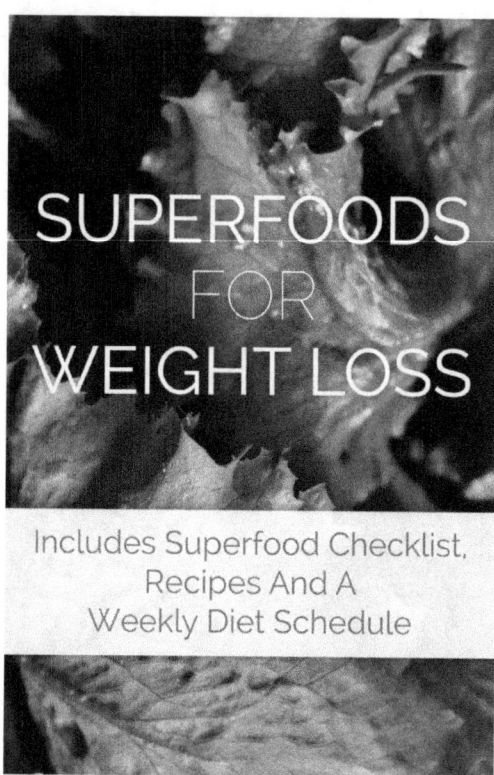

Learn about simple superfoods that can not only help you los weight but also, strengthen your body and improve mental performance. These foods are packed with nutrients, antioxidants and often have amazing side bonuses – like cancer fighting agents. Includes a superfood checklist and an easy to follow diet schedule.

>> You Can Download This Free Report By Clicking Here <<

FREE GIFT

Kindle 5 Star Books

Free Kindle 5 Star Book Club Membership

Join Other Kindle 5 Star Members Who Are Getting Private Access To Weekly Free Kindle Book Promotions

Get free Kindle books

Stay connected:

Join our Facebook group

Follow Kindle 5 Star on Twitter

Also, if you want to receive updates on Jessica David's new books, free promotions and Kindle countdown deals sign up to her New Release Mailing List.

TABLE OF CONTENTS

INTRODUCTION

The coconut has been used for centuries throughout the tropics for food and medicine, among many other practical uses. In fact, medicinally, it has also been used to treat everything from scabies (an infection caused by the human itch mite), baldness, tumors, ulcers, colds, and dry skin, among other ailments. In Indian culture, for instance, coconut oil has been used by women to improve their hair. It has also been claimed to improve eyes sight and help the sick.

Yet due to its high saturated fat content, coconut oil has been demonized as bad for good health when used with food. In more recent years, however, a better understanding of the types of fat that cause poor cardiovascular health has lead researchers to revise their view of coconut oil. It appears that the medium chain saturated fatty acids in coconut oil can actually be good for your health. It has been observed that in countries like Sri Lanka, where the diet is rich in coconut oil, has less cardiovascular disease than what is typically seen in the West, indicating that coconut oil may not be as unhealthy as previously believed. Some of the benefit may come from the fact that the body can dissolve medium chain fatty acids, unlike the saturated fat made of long chain fatty acids, which does lead to cardiovascular problems. Among the other health benefits of coconut oil use, there are many. Coconut oil has been used for decades in lotion in the US. For centuries it has also been used as topically in the tropics, used to treat dry skin. Coconut oil also has anti-bacterial properties such that it can also help those with ulcers. One study has also shown that coconut oil can also help reduce the amount of protein lost in hair. Slowly, research is demonstrating that the centuries-old use of coconut oil does have a great amount of health benefits.

CHAPTER 1

Coconut Oil Defined

The Coconut and Coconut Oil

Coconut oil comes from the coconut (Cocos nucifera); a fruit that grows on the coconut palm. The exact origins of the coconut tree are uncertain, they were thought to have originated in India and Australia, although other scientists think that they may have started in the Americas. Regardless of where they originated, coconuts are considered to be the largest seed plant. Coconuts, scientifically speaking, are drupes and have three main parts — these consist of a smooth exocarp, a fibrous middle part called the mesocarp, and hard woody part called the endocarp, which surrounds the seed. The seed contains the small plant which could grow into another adult coconut tree, under the right conditions. The round, brown part of the coconut, that is typically seen at the grocery store, is the endocarp section.

Although scientifically a drupe, coconuts can be generically classified as a fruit, seed and a nut. It can be considered a fruit because it contains a seed. It can be considered a seed because it houses the reproductive part of the plant. It can be considered a nut because it is a fruit with one seed. The three dark spots or "eyes" located at one end of the coconut is where the new coconut begins to germinate, if the coconut were placed under the right conditions for growing (i.e., placed in the ground, ideally with the exocarp still intact, and adequately watered). The exocarp of the coconut, which is seen when it is growing on a tree, can be many different colors including green, yellow, or brown. Some of these different colors are related to the stage of development that the coconut is in. For instance, the green exocarp is seen in immature coconuts.

There are several varieties of coconuts, including; the coconut, double coconut, dwarf orange coconut, dwarf green coconut, Maypan coconut, Golden Malay coconut, Nawassi coconut, the Fiji dwarf, the dwarf Green coconut and the King coconut, among others. Coconuts live in various tropical and semi-tropical areas around the world, including; Malaysia, Indonesia, India, Sri Lanka, Hawaii, various southern states in the US (Florida, the Carolinas and Georgia), Puerto Rico, Madagascar, Belize, Palau, Tanzania and Papau New Guinea, among other places. They tend to grow in areas 25 degrees to the north and 25 degrees south of the equator.

The coconut palm can grow to be 100 feet tall, it's leaves can be quite extensive as well. Some of the largest palm leaves were seen in a palm in Africa, that was about 82 feet long and 4 feet wide.

The whole coconut, from the exocarp to the coconut water is used in various ways. The fibrous exocarp is used to make fibers, the coconut milk, the white meat of the coconut can be eaten and the water in the coconut can be drank. The trunk can be used in the construction of buildings. The hard outer brown part can be used in various ways, including making musical instruments. Also, the leaves of the coconut tree are used for thatch or can be woven into baskets, clothing and mats.

Besides having many practical and material uses, the coconut has a religious or cultural significance as well in various parts of the world. For instance, in India the coconut, along with incense sticks and flowers has traditionally been used in worshipping a Hindu god. The coconut itself symbolizes God; the Sanskrit word for coconut, Sriphala, means God's fruit.

In the Hawaiian Islands, the coconut tree has been used to create everything from clothing, to drums, to containers for food, to sennit (rope yarn), among many other things. Additionally, it appears in a Hawaiian legend where it symbolizes a link to the divine, to ancestors, and to the original home of the native Hawaiian people, in the Asian South Pacific.

How Coconut Oil is Produced

Coconut oil is made from the white meat, or endosperm, of the coconut. There are various types of coconut oil, these include; refined, hydrogenated, fractionated (aka liquid or MCT) and virgin coconut oil, depending on how it is manufactured.

Refined coconut oil can be made by drying the endosperm of the coconut in a variety of ways, including; sun-drying, smoke-drying, drying in a kiln or using a mixture, or a variation of these methods. After the meat is dried it is called copra. The end product made from copra is refined, bleached and deodorized. The oil is bleached by using bleaching clays. The deodorization occurs by using steam. The oil is also processed by using sodium hydroxide to rid the oil of free fatty acids; this allows the product to have a longer shelf life. The above process is the most common manner in which coconut oil is manufactured.

Hydrogenated coconut oil is made by adding hydrogens to the coconut oil in order to make it solid at room temperature. This would be more of an issue in warmer, tropical climates as the melting point of coconut oil is 76 degrees F. Most of the fats in coconut oil are medium chain fatty acids that are nonetheless, saturated fats. Saturated fats already have lots of hydrogen attached to them, this is what makes them "saturated" so there is not a lot of hydrogen that gets added to the oil. However, this process of hydrogenation creates trans fats. Due to health concerns, foods containing trans fats have been banned in some European countries and the US. Thus, hydrogenated coconut oil is not something typically seen in the US.

Fractionated coconut oil has the lauric acid removed from it, which allows it to remain a liquid when at a lower temperature. Lauric acid is a medium chain fatty acid contained in coconut oil, which may help to give this oil its health benefits.

Virgin coconut oil is oil that is technically less processed than other coconut oils. Unlike the olive oil industry, there is no industry standard for the manufacturing or labelling of virgin coconut oil, so this label may even be found on products that are not virgin coconut oil. Commercially, consumers may even find virgin coconut oil labeled as extra virgin, but this label appears to not mean much due to the lack of an industry-wide standard.

Virgin coconut oil can be made by either of two methods; the wet-milling or the expeller-pressing method. In the wet-milling process, the coconut meat is pressed out so that the coconut "milk" is removed. This milk is then further processed so that the water is removed from the oil in the milk. The water can be removed from the milk by various methods including centrifugation, refrigeration, fermentation, boiling, and enzymes. In the expeller-pressing method, the coconut meat is dried, thus making it copra. The copra is then pressed so that the oil is removed from it. Using this method it is easy for mass production.

Coconut oil can also be made at home by using five medium to large coconuts. These nuts are cut open and then the white meat, or kernel, is removed. The kernel is then cut into small pieces and placed into a blender with 2 cups of water. The mixture is blended until smooth. This mixture is then put through a sieve to remove the solids and the resulting liquid is allowed to sit for a minimum of 24 hours. The resulting cream is skimmed off the top, as the cream and the water separate, the cream can then be placed in a heavy and deep pot and cooked. The pot is placed on medium heat — this will create the oil and also curdled cream. The curdled cream is moved to the side of the pot and the coconut oil can then be poured out into a separate container, as it cooks out from the cream. The cooking process should continue until there is no more oil coming from the cream. Five coconut can yield 1 cup of coconut oil. Also it is important to cook until a low flame so that the phytonutrients in the oil are not harmed.

Thus, from the coconut comes a nutritious food and oil which contain some important nutrients that are listed below.

Nutritional Benefits of Coconut per 100 mg[51][52]

Energy	354kCal
Saturated Fat	29.70 g
Monounsaturated Fat	1.43
Carbohydrates	15.23 g
Dietary Fiber	9.0 g
Sugars	6.23 g
Protein	3.33 g
Cholesterol	0 mg
Folates	26 μg (micrograms)
Vitamin K	0.2 μg
Vitamin C	3.3. mg
Vitamin E	0.24 mg
Vitamin A	0 IU (International Units)
Thiamin	0.066 mg
Niacin	0.540 mg
Riboflavin	0.020 mg
Pyridoxine (Vitamin B6)	0.054 mg

Pantothenic Acid	0.300 mg
Potassium	356 mg
Sodium	20mg
Zinc	1.10 mg
Calcium	14 mg
Iron	2.43 mg
Copper	0.435 mg
Manganese	1.5 mg
Magnesium	32 mg
Selenium	10.1 µg
Phosphorus	113 mg
Phytosterols	47 mg
Beta-carotene	0 µg

Just as coconuts contain a lot of important nutrients, so does the oil which comes from coconuts contains important fatty acids that research has indicated can be good for health. Below are the nutrients found in coconut oil.

Nutritional Benefits of Coconut Oil per 100g

Energy	862 kCal
Total Fat	100.00 g

Total Saturated Fatty

Acids	86.5 g

Total Monounsaturated Fatty

Acids   5.8 g

Total Polyunsaturated Fatty

Acids	1.8 g
Carbohydrates	0 g
Dietary Fiber	0 g
Sugars	0 g
Protein	0 g
Cholesterol	0 g
Folates	0 µg
Vitamin K	0.5 µg
Vitamin C	0 mg
Vitamin E	0.09 mg
Vitamin A	0 IU (International Units)
Thiamin	0 mg
Niacin	0 mg
Riboflavin	0 mg
Pyridoxine (Vitamin B6)	0 mg

Potassium	0 mg
Sodium	0mg
Zinc	0 mg
Calcium	0 mg
Iron	0.04 mg
Magnesium	0 mg
Phosphorus	0 mg

CHAPTER 2

Coconut Oil for Weight Loss

Generally, there tends to be little scientific research performed on natural products. Yet the few studies that have been conducted to determine if coconut oil does help with weight loss in humans seem to indicate that coconut oil may help with weight loss. This may be due to the fact that coconut oil has medium chain fatty acids, which are not stored in adipose (fat) cells in the body. It must be said that no firm scientific conclusions can be drawn from only a few research studies, however. Much more research would need to be conducted before anything definitive can be said about whether coconut oil could be used to help with weight loss. Health experts do emphasize, that using coconut oil is not a substitute for eating a healthy diet and getting plenty of exercise, in order to lose weight.

The Malaysian Study

A study published in 2011 and conducted in Malaysia looked at the use of virgin coconut oil in 20 obese but otherwise healthy male and female volunteers. The study subjects were mostly female-13 females and 7 males-and had a body mass index, or BMI, of equal to or over 25kg/m2 . The subjects were therefore considered obese. During the study the volunteers consumed 30 mL each day of virgin coconut oil in three separate doses 30 minutes before a meal. The coconut oil was provided by a local agricultural company and contained no additives or preservatives.

The results of the study indicated some amount of loss in waist circumference. In other words, some of the study volunteers had lost a few centimeters off their waist. All the male volunteers had a waist circumference over 90 cm at the start of the study. The female volunteers had a waist circumference of over 80 cm, except for one volunteer with a circumference of 77 cm at the start of the study. The results showed that after looking at different variables being measured in the study volunteers only the waist circumference was reduced. There was an average decrease of about 3 cm, +/- about 5 cm, or a reduction of less than one percent. But only in the male volunteers was there a reduction that researchers considered statistically significant. Other variables looked at in the study, like HDL (high-density lipoprotein), total cholesterol, and FFM (fat free mass), and body weight, liver function, electrolytes, among others, did not show a significant increase or decrease. (8)

Other Potential Health Effects of Coconut Oil

Other studies, often in countries where coconut production and consumption are high, have indicated that there are various potential health benefits to using coconut oil. Below are summaries of some of the studies and their results.

A Study in India

In 2004, another study performed in rats, showed that virgin coconut oil appeared to reduce the levels of lipids in tissues and serum, among other benefits. The researchers fed the coconut oil to the animals for 45 days. They then took and analyzed blood samples and noted that there was a reduction in lipids. Specifically, the level of triglycerides, phospholipids, total cholesterol, low density lipoprotein and very low density lipoprotein. There was also an increase in the high density lipoprotein, the so-called good cholesterol. The researchers suggested that the polyphenols in the oil may be the reason for these health effects. (31)

A Study in Brazil (32)

A study in Brazil indicated that, in contrast to the Malaysian study, obese women could have a reduction in their waist circumference by using coconut oil. Study participants in this experiment, were women with a waist circumference over 88 cm. They were split into two groups. One group took dietary supplements of 30mL of coconut oil daily while the other group took supplements of 30mL of soybean oil daily over a 12 week timeframe. The study participants were told to eat a low calorie diet and to walk 50 minutes each day. The results of the study indicated that both groups experienced a reduction in BMI. Yet only the group given coconut oil experienced a decrease in the waist circumference and no dyslipidemia, or a high level of fats in the blood.

A Study in Thailand (33)

In a 2010 study in rats, it was demonstrated that use of virgin coconut oil could moderately reduce inflammation in rats with ear edema induced by ethyl phenylpropiolate, as well as in paw edema induced by carrageenin and arachidonic acid. There was also an anti-pyretic (anti-fever) effect in hyperthermia induced by yeast as well as a pain reducing effect seen in acetic acid-induce writhing (wiggling due to pain).

As this study was performed in rats more research would have to be done to determine if the same effects would occur in humans.

A study in Malaysia in rats

An early 2015 study in mice looked at the antioxidant and anti-stress effects of virgin coconut oil. The researchers used two types of tests to create stress, the forced swim test and the cold restraint test. In the forced swim test, the mice were divided into three groups. One group was given virgin coconut oil, another group was given diazepam (an antidepressant), and the untreated group was given saline for 6 days. On day 6 the animals were allowed to swim to get used to the exercise. Then, on day 7 the time that the mice swam freely and the time that they just floated in an upright position in the water with little movement was measured, after they had been in the water for three minutes. The mice were then euthanized and the levels of stress-related chemicals found in their livers were analyzed.

Another set of mice were subjected to the chronic cold restraint stress test. In this experiment 32 mice were divided into four groups. One group was the control, which included untreated mice who were not subjected to stress, another group included mice who were stressed but were untreated and given saline. A third group of mice were stressed and were given diazepam and another group was stressed and given virgin coconut oil. For 7 days the mice in the untreated control group, the positive control group (those given diazepam) and the virgin coconut oil group were placed in conditions of 4 degree C cold restraint for one hour. Afterwards these mice were euthanized and various chemicals in their bodies were analyzed.

The researchers found that the mice treated with diazepam or virgin coconut oil and subjected to the forced swim test had less immobility time. Immobility time was an indication of depression in the animals. Therefore, the animals with less immobility had less depression. Animals untreated by diazepam or virgin coconut oil had the longest immobility time. Similar results were seen with the cold restraint test. Mice given diazepam or virgin coconut oil had, among other things, lower adrenal gland weights, which is an indication of decreased stress, compared to untreated mice in the study. Between diazepam and coconut oil, the coconut oil had the greater anti-depressant effect, based on the results of this study.

Therefore, consumption of virgin coconut oil appeared to decrease stress in mice. Again, more studies would have to be performed to see if this effect could also be seen in humans. (34)

Breast Cancer Study in Malaysia

In another study performed in Malaysia, 60 breast cancer patients participated in an experiment to determine if ingestion of coconut oil had an effect on their quality of life. (The study authors noted that breast cancer is the most common type of cancer affecting women in Malaysia and that this cancer can negatively affect quality of life for patients dealing with it.) The patient in the study were in stage III and IV of their cancer and were undergoing six cycles of chemotherapy. The authors noted that these volunteers were experiencing negative symptoms due to their treatment such as loss of appetite, loss of sexual desire, hair loss, pain, depression, among other problems. The control groups were not given virgin coconut oil, while the intervention group did receive it. The results showed that those given coconut oil had an improved quality of life. The intervention group had a reduction in certain symptoms like loss of appetite, sleep difficulties, dyspnea and fatigue, among other improvements. Overall, the use of coconut oil had a positive effect on the quality of life of the patients who received it. (35)

Study in New Zealand

A study in New Zealand, published in 2003, did not look at the health benefits of coconut oil directly, but it did examine whether fatty acids and monoglycerides had an impact on Helicobacter pylori, or H. pylori, the stomach bacteria responsible for creating ulcers, among other ailments. (This relates to health claims about coconut oil since some have stated that it can be used to treat ulcers. Also, coconut oil contains a sizeable amount of medium chain fatty acids.) Researchers exposed these bacteria in vitro (meaning in a Petri dish) to various fatty acids, including lauric acid which is found in coconut oil, and monoglycerides at different pH levels. The experiment indicated that the H. pylori bacteria died as a result of such exposure. They also died when exposed to monoglycerides. Death of the bacteria started slowly but then grew to about a 90% death rate after extended exposure to the fatty acids. Even small increase in the concentrations of fatty acids had a large impact on the number of bacteria killed. The potency of the fatty acids was dependent on the pH, however. A change in potency was observed with the decrease of the pH. The potency of the monoglycerides was not pH dependent, however. Moreover, research suggests that H. pylori, unlike antibiotics, is not resistant to fatty acids.

The reason why the H. pylori dies in the presence of the fatty acids and the monoglycerides is not certain. It has been theorized that it may be because the cell membrane of the bacteria becomes permeable under certain pH conditions, allowing the fatty acids enter and, ultimately, destroy the cell. More studies are needed to determine why fatty acids have this effect on H. pylori. Monoglycerides might be able to enter and destroy the H. pylori cells because they can form micelles (spheres).

The results of this study suggest that since coconut oil does contain fatty acids, this may explain the anti-ulcer effect of coconut oil, which some claim. But multiple studies using human subjects would need to be performed to determine if coconut oil really can help treat stomach ulcers.

CHAPTER 3

Summary of Health Benefits of Coconut Oil

Much research still needs to be done to assess what the real health benefits of coconut oil are. But the studies that has been done suggest that coconut oil may be beneficial for certain conditions. For instance, it may help to reduce the negative symptoms associated with chemotherapy treatments, to decrease the symptoms of depression in mice, to reduce inflammation in mice, and also to reduce the waistline of obese individuals. There have been other claims about coconut oil including that it can help with HIV, head lice, diabetes, Crohn's disease, but there does not seem to be enough evidence to suggest that this is the case. (*38*)

CHAPTER 4

Drink Recipes Using Coconut Oil

Here is a sampling of some of the ways that coconut oil can be used in drinks. No overt health benefit is being claimed by including these recipes.

Banana Smoothie (10)

Ingredients:

- One banana
- About 1/2 cup of orange juice
- 3 tablespoons of liquid virgin coconut oil
- 1 tablespoon of coconut cream concentrate
- 3 tablespoons of organic whole milk vanilla yogurt
- 3 ice cubes

Directions:

1. Except for the coconut oil, mix all the ingredients together into a blender. Add the coconut oil in by drops and then a steady stream.

2. (Frozen strawberries might also be used in this smoothie.)

3. After the ingredients are thoroughly blended. Enjoy.

London Fog *(11)*

Ingredients:

- Eight ounces of hot Earl Grey tea
- 1.5 tablespoons of coconut oil
- 1/4cup of almond milk or some other non-dairy milk
- 1/4of vanilla extract
- Sweeten to taste with the favorite sweetener

Directions:

1. Place all the ingredients into a blender.

2. Blend on high for 1 minute.

3. The consistency of the drink should be frothy like a latte. (Another name for a London Fog is Earl Grey latte.)

Healthy Key Lime Pie Milkshake (15)

Ingredients:

- 2 tablespoons of key lime juice
- 2 tablespoons of coconut oil
- 1 cup of light coconut milk
- 1 teaspoon of key lime zest
- 1 ripe frozen banana
- 1 teaspoon of agave nectar
- 1 teaspoon of pure vanilla extract
- 2 tablespoons of graham crackers

Directions:

1. Combine all the ingredients into a blender and pulse them until the mixture is smooth.

2. Pour into a glass and top with a dairy or soy-based whipped cream. Sprinkle additional graham crackers on top of the drink and top with a lime slice.

Strawberry Lime Shake (16)

Ingredients:

- 1 1/2 cups of coconut milk
- 1 tablespoon freshly squeezed lime juice
- 1 tablespoon of coconut oil (optional)
- 1 10-ounce package of strawberries, frozen

Directions:

1. Place all ingredients in a vitamix, a type of blender, and puree on high until smooth

2. Serve!

Coconut Mango Banana Smoothie (17)

Ingredients:

- 1 tablespoon extra virgin coconut oil
- 1 cup unsweetened almond milk/coconut milk blend (or another non-dairy milk)
- 1 organic sliced mango
- 1 organic banana peeled
- 1 tablespoon maple syrup (or any other sweetener of your choice honey, Stevia, raw sugar, dates, etc.)
- 1 teaspoon of vanilla extract
- 1 handful of ice
- 1/2 tablespoons of unsweetened coconut flakes for topping, optional

Directions:

1. Put all the ingredients into a blender and puree them until smooth and creamy.
2. Serve the drink immediately.
3. Sprinkle coconut flakes on top, if desired.

Joker Juice Smoothies *(18)*

Ingredients:

- 10 ounces of mixed berries
- 1/2 cup of any kind of milk (cow's, soy, almond, etc.)
- 2 bananas
- 1 orange (peeled)
- 1 tablespoon of coconut oil
- 2 tablespoons of honey

Directions:

1. Mix all ingredients in a blender (preferably a Vitamix). Blend on high until the mix is smooth.

2. Enjoy the drink!

Double Matcha Green Tea Blast (20)

Ingredients:

- 1/2 frozen banana
- 5 ice cubes
- 1 teaspoon melted coconut oil
- 1 cup of half and half
- 1/2 teaspoon of cinnamon

One tea bag of double matcha green tea powder (The tea can come in small discs that are cut open. The contents of the disc are then placed in the drink.)

Directions:

1. Blend all the ingredients until they are smooth.

2. Serve!

Hot Cocoa That's Exploding with Superfoods (21)

Ingredients:

- 2 cups of vanilla almond milk
- 1 tablespoon (heaping, not leveled off) raw cocoa
- 1 tablespoon of coconut oil
- 1 tablespoon of raw honey
- 1/2 teaspoon of cinnamon

Directions:

1. Heat the almond milk until it is almost to a boil. Mix all the ingredients together in a blender or in a vitamix for 1 minute.

Keto Pumpkin Spice Latte (22)

Ingredients:

- Pumpkin Spice tea bags
- Cinnamon
- 1-3 teaspoons of coconut oil (can also use ghee or butter)
- Water
- Stevia to taste
- Salt (a pinch)

Directions:

1. Brew a mug of pumpkin spice tea. Allow it to steep for a minimum of 5 minutes for taste.
2. Add 1 to 3 tablespoons of coconut oil to a blender.
3. Pour tea, without the tea bag, into the blender.
4. Add salt and Stevia.
5. Blend the mixture until it is creamy and frothy.
6. Pour the drink back into the same mug the tea was in and sprinkle with cinnamon.

Hot Chocolate Zen *(23)*

Ingredients:

- 1/2 cup of almond milk (along with 1/2 cup of water warmed up on the stove)
- 1 tablespoon of coconut oil
- 1/2 teaspoon of raw maca powder
- 1/2 teaspoon of tumeric
- 1/2 teaspoon of maple syrup
- 1 tablespoon of raw cocoa powder
- 3 dashes of cinnamon
- Pinch of Cayenne
- Pinch of Sea salt

Directions:

1. Use a blender to thoroughly blend all the ingredients.
2. Enjoy!

Chocolate Banana Wonderland Breakfast Smoothie (62)

Ingredients:

- 1 banana, unfrozen or frozen
- 1 teaspoon of organic cinnamon
- 1 cup unsweetened almond or coconut milk
- 2 tablespoons of raw organic cacao powder
- 1 tablespoon of organic virgin coconut oil
- 2 tablespoons of natural peanut butter
- Ice cubes

Directions:

1. Put all the ingredients into a blender.

2. Blend the ingredients on medium to high, until the mixture is foamy. The ice cubes can be added during the mixing if the blender can deal with them, if not then add them at the end.

CHAPTER 5

Coconut Oil in Food Recipes

Here is a sampling of some of the ways that coconut oil can be used in food. No overt health benefit is being claimed by including these recipes.

Roast Chicken with Coconut Oil *(14)*

Ingredients:

- 1 whole chicken
- 1 small yellow onion, quartered
- 1 stalk of celery
- 4 garlic cloves, halved
- 1/4cup of melted coconut oil
- 1/2 teaspoon of garlic powder
- 1/2 cup of chicken stock (water can be used or a combination of the two)
- 1 1/2 tablespoon of corn starch
- 2 tablespoons of water
- Salt to taste
- Black pepper to taste
- 1/4cup of melted butter

Directions:

1. Preheat the oven to 425 degrees F.

2. Take out the giblets and clean the chicken in warm to hot tap water. Thoroughly dry.

3. Season the cavity of the chicken with salt and pepper liberally. Then stuff the cavity with onion, garlic and celery.

4. Brush the coconut oil and melted butter over the chicken. Season the outside of the chicken with salt, garlic powder and pepper.

5. Place in a 9 x 13 glass baking pan or a roasting pan.

6. Roast the chicken for 11 minutes at 425 degrees F.

7. Decrease the heat to 350 degrees F and baste the chicken. Roast the chicken for 1 hour or until the juices are clear after sticking the chicken between the thigh and the leg. Baste the chicken every 10-15 minutes. Stop the basting for the last 10 minutes. To speed up cooking the temperature can be increased to 375 degrees F during the last 30 minutes.

8. Pour the juices from the pan into a saucepan. Add water or chicken stock. Adjust the richness of the sauce by adding more or less chicken stock or water.

9. Add corn starch to the water and then whisk the corn starch into the gravy to get the right thickness. Add more stock if that is needed. Continue to whisk and boil the mixture until it has thickened.

10. Serve the gravy with the roasted chicken.

~ ❖ ~

Superfood Candy Cups *(12)*

Ingredients:

- 3 tablespoons of virgin coconut oil
- 1 tablespoon raw maca powder
- 1/2 cup of unsweetened almond butter or sunflower seed butter
- 1 teaspoon of ground cinnamon
- 4 ounces of chopped unsweetened chocolate
- A pinch of salt
- 1/4cup of honey and 1 tablespoon of honey or maple syrup (to be used separately)

Directions:

(For the Filling)

1. In a bowl mix the almond butter or sunflower seed butter, 1 tablespoon of honey or maple syrup, cinnamon, maca powder and salt. Stir the ingredients until a thick dough is created. If the doughy consistency does not happen, then add more maca powder.

2. Roll the dough into 16 small balls; use one teaspoon of dough for each ball.

3. Then flatten each ball into a pancake shape. (The little dough that is left over can be rolled into a larger ball to snack on later.)

(For the Chocolate Coating)

1. Place the chocolate, the rest of the 1/4cup of honey, and coconut oil in a small pot over low heat.

2. Stir the mixture constantly until it is smooth and fully melted.

3. Line a mini-muffin tin with 16 paper liners. Spoon in enough of the chocolate mixture to coat the bottom. (Do not use all the chocolate mixture.)

4. Place the chocolate in the tin in the freezer for 5-10 minutes until the chocolate is firm.

5. Place a small "pancake" of filling into each cup. Cover the patty with the rest of the chocolate (so that it resembles a Reese's peanut butter cup).

6. Sprinkle the tops of the candy cups with cacao nibs and place the candy in the freezer until it sets-for about 30 minutes.

7. Store the candies in an air tight container in the freezer or refrigerator.

8. Note: Cocoa powder can be substituted for the maca powder and maple syrup can be substituted for honey.

~ ❖ ~

Banana Bread with Coffee and Coconut Oil (13)

Ingredients:

- 1 cup of whole wheat flour
- 1 cup of unbleached all-purpose flour
- 1 teaspoon of baking soda
- 1/4teaspoon of ground cinnamon
- 1 teaspoon of sea salt
- 3/4 cup grade B maple syrup, room temperature
- 4 large overly ripe bananas
- 1/2 cup of hot coffee
- 2 tablespoons of ground flax seed
- 1/4cup of melted, unrefined, organic coconut oil

Directions:

1. Preheat the oven to 350 degrees F. Add oil to an 8 x 4 1/2 x 2 1/2-inch loaf pan. The loaf pan should ideally be made from glass or enamel cast iron.

2. In a medium bowl, mix together the flax powder with the hot coffee or water using a whisk. It should have a gelantinous consistency. Set aside.

3. In a large bowl, mix together the wheat and all-purpose flours along with the cinnamon, salt and baking soda.

4. In the medium bowl, add the bananas and mash them very well. Stir in the maple syrup, coconut oil and reserved flax mixture.

5. Combine the banana mixture to the dry ingredients and mix until smooth.

6. Pour the batter into the lightly oiled pan. Bake for 75 minutes, or until it is cooked through. This can be tested by inserting a toothpick into the bread and it comes out clean, with few or no crumbs on it.

7. Allow the banana bread to cool on the rack for 20 minutes before turning it out of the pan. Allow the bread to cool completely before slicing it.

50/50 Olive Oil/Coconut Oil Blend Healthy Chicken Stir Fry (24)

Ingredients:

- 1 tablespoon oil blend
- 1/2 cups sliced carrots
- 2 teaspoons of minced fresh garlic
- 2 teaspoons of minced fresh ginger
- 2 teaspoons of hoisin sauce
- 2 tablespoons of soy sauce
- 1 cup of cooked chicken
- 1 bunch of scallions, chopped
- 1 cup of sliced mushrooms
- 1/2 cups of broccoli, chopped

Directions:

1. Heat the oil in a large frying pan.

2. Add the garlic, ginger and carrots.

3. Stirring quickly, cook the ingredients in a pan until they are tender. Add the chicken, soy sauce and hoisin sauce. Continue stirring for about 3-4 minutes. Add the scallions, mushrooms and broccoli. Cook for about 2 minutes and then serve.

Salmon with Coconut Sauce (25)

Ingredients:

- 4 tablespoons of coconut oil, divided
- 1 teaspoon of fennel seeds
- 1 teaspoon of cardamom seeds
- 1 teaspoon of brown mustard seeds
- 1 tablespoon of finely chopped ginger
- 1 tablespoon of ground coriander, along with 1/2 teaspoon to season the salmon
- 1/4to 1/2 cup of chopped tomatoes
- 2 (6 ounce) salmon fillets
- 1 cup of coconut milk
- Salt and black pepper to taste

Directions:

(For the Sauce)

1. Put 2 tablespoons of coconut oil into a large pan over medium heat. Add ginger.

2. Saute for 30 minutes. Add the fennel seeds, brown mustard seeds, cardamom seeds, and ground coriander.

3. Cook for 10 seconds.

4. Add tomatoes. Cook for 3 minutes, stirring well.

5. Pour in the coconut milk. Simmer for about 15 minutes, until the sauce is thick.

6. Add seasoning to taste. If needed, add salt and pepper.

(For the Salmon)

1. Heat the rest of the coconut oil (2 tablespoons worth) in a non-stick pan over medium heat.

2. When hot, season the salmon fillets using 1/2 teaspoon of coriander, a pinch of salt and pepper.

3. Sear the fillets on both sides, for 7-8 minutes for each side.

4. Place the salmon on a plate and ladle the sauce over the fillets.

~ ❖ ~

Super Easy Tandoori Chicken *(26)*

Ingredients:

- 4 chicken thighs (skin-on, bone-in)
- 1 cup of full-fat Greek yogurt (or full fat coconut milk)
- 1 tablespoon of kosher salt
- 1 tablespoon of tandoori seasoning
- 1 tablespoon of coconut oil (or choice of fat)
- Juice from 1/2 lemon

Directions:

1. Remove excess pieces of fat from the thighs.

2. Season the chicken parts evenly and stick them into the bowl.

3. In a different bowl, place the tandoori seasoning and yogurt.

4. Add the lemon juice and mix well.

5. After the marinade is complete, then spoon it over the salted chicken.

6. Rub the marinade into the chicken using your hands.

7. Cover the bowl using plastic wrap and refrigerate for 4-8 hours.

8. Preheat the oven to 375 degree F, on convention roast setting. Set the oven to 400 degrees F for a non-convection oven.

9. Put a wire rack on a foil-lined baking sheet. Grease the rack with coconut oil by simply dipping a paper towel in oil.

10. Place the chicken on the rack with the skin side down.

11. Put the tray in the oven for 40 minutes.

12. Flip the chicken half way between the baking time.

13. The meat is done when the juices run clear after the chicken has been stabbed by a skewer and small charred bits are on the chicken.

~ ❖ ~

Paleo Coconut Chicken (27)

Ingredients:

- 1 pound skinless and boneless chicken breasts
- 1/4cup of coconut flour
- 1 egg
- 1/4unsweetened shredded coconut
- 1/2 cup garlic powder
- 2 tablespoons of coconut oil
- Crushed red pepper and sea salt to taste

Directions:

1. Mix coconut flour, shredded coconut, red pepper, sea salt, garlic powder in a bowl.

2- Beat the egg using a separate bowl.

3. Take the chicken breast and dip it into the beaten egg. Roll the chicken in the dry mixture until it is fully coated.

4. Heat a frying pan over medium heat and add coconut oil until the pan is hot.

5. Pan-fry chicken until it is cooked all the way through. If you have a large chicken breast then the outside might full cook before the inside is done. If this is the case, then move the chicken from the pan and put in the oven at 350 degree F for 5-10 minutes.

6. Alternatively, the chicken may be cooked entirely in the oven at 400 degree F for 25 minutes.

7. You may serve this with sweet potato fries.

Coconut Oil Chocolate Chip Cookies *(28)*

Ingredients:

- 1 1/2 cups of All-purpose flour
- 1/2 teaspoon baking soda
- 1/2 teaspoon baking powder
- 1/4teaspoon of salt
- 1/2 cup of dark brown sugar
- 1/4cup of granulated sugar
- 1/2 cup of coconut oil at room temperature
- 1 teaspoon of vanilla extract
- 1 cup of semi-sweet chocolate morsels
- 1 egg

Directions:

1. Whisk together the baking soda, baking powder, salt and flour, in a small bowl. Set it aside.

2. Cream the coconut oil and sugars using an electric mixer. Do this in a medium sized bowl. Cream until the mixture is fluffy and light.

3. Add the egg and vanilla to the bowl until everything is combined.

4. Gradually mix in the dry ingredients with the wet ingredients. Mix until everything is well blended. Stir in the chocolate chips.

5. Refrigerate the dough for at least 2 hours. It can be kept overnight as well.

6. Preheat the oven to 350 degrees F. Line the cookie sheet with parchment paper.

7. Scoop rounded tablespoons full of dough onto the cookie sheet, setting them two inches apart.

8. Bake for 7-9 minutes or until the edges are slightly brown. Move the cookies to a wire rack to cool all the way.

Blueberry Muffins with Flax Seed and Coconut Oil (29)

Ingredients:

- 3 cups of flour
- 4 teaspoons of baking powder
- 1/3 cup of flax meal
- 1 teaspoon of salt
- 2/3 cup of coconut oil
- 2/3 cup of milk
- 2 large eggs
- 2 cups of blueberries
- 1 teaspoon of vanilla
- For the icing: 1/2 cup of confectioners sugar
- 1 ounce of cream cheese
- 1 tablespoon increments of milk to thin the icing to the consistency desired.

Directions:

1. Preheat the oven to 375 degrees F.

2. Use paper liners or oil the muffin tin cups.

3. Whisk the dry ingredients (excluding the blueberries) together in a large bowl.

4. Mix the wet ingredients together in a medium bowl. (The milk and oil may need to be warmed to lukewarm, so that the coconut oil is in liquid form.)

5. Place the wet ingredients in with the dry ingredients and mix with an electric mixer. The result should be a stiff dough.

6. Fold the blueberries carefully into the mixture after it has been well blended. Try to not break the berries.

7. Spoon the dough into the muffin tin cups.

8. Bake the muffins for 18-20 minutes, until an inserted toothpick comes out clean and the tops are a nice light brown.

9. Take from the oven and wait for the muffins to cool so that they can be handled. Go along the edges of the blueberries with a knife to separate them from the sides of the muffin tin.

10. Continue with cooling the muffins on wire racks.

11. For the icing, place the cream cheese and sugar in a small, deep bowl. Mix the ingredients on low speed until the sugar is thoroughly incorporated into the cream cheese.

12. Increase the speed of the mixer to medium and, in small increments, add the milk until the icing is smooth and has the desired consistency.

13. Making sure the muffins are cool, place the icing on them.

~ ❖ ~

Coconut Flour Bread (30)

Ingredients:

- 1/2 cup of coconut flour
- 1/4teaspoon of baking soda
- 1/4teaspoon of Celtic sea salt
- 1/2 cup of coconut oil, melted or unsweetened almond milk
- 6 eggs

Directions:

1. Preheat the oven to 350 degrees F.
2. Sift the dry ingredients together in a medium bowl.
3. Slowly add the wet ingredients to dry ingredients. Stir until the mixture is smooth.
4. Grease a small bread pan and fill 2/3 of the way full with the batter.
5. Bake in the oven for 40-50 minutes or until the toothpick emerges clean.

Swedish Chocolate Balls *(61)*

Ingredients:

- Four cups of rolled oats
- 1 1/4cup of raw sugar, can use raw cane sugar
- 1/2 cup of unsweetened cocoa, can use Ghirardelli cocoa
- 3/4 cup of grass-fed butter (meaning the cows from which the butter comes were fed on grass)
- 2 tablespoons of coconut oil, can use Tropical Traditions
- 2 tablespoons of ground coffee
- 1 teaspoon of pure vanilla extract
- Half of a chocolate baking bar
- Coconut flakes

Directions:

1. Melt the coconut oil and the butter together in a pan.

2. Melt the half bar of baking chocolate in a separate pot on low heat.

3. Place the coconut flakes into a small bowl.

4. In a large bowl place the rolled oats, sugar, unsweetened cocoa, butter (melted), coconut oil (melted), the ground coffee, vanilla extract and the melted chocolate bar.

5. Combine the ingredients together using a mixing spoon. Don't be afraid to use your hands, if needed, to mix the ingredients.

6. Combine until all the ingredients are well mixed and then take some dough and roll it into a golf ball-sized ball. Roll the chocolate ball in the small bowl of coconut.

7. Place it on a baking sheet.

8. Do this until all the dough has been used up.

9. The chocolate balls are now ready to eat or they may be placed in the refrigerator for approximately 2 hours and then eaten.

~ ❖ ~

CHAPTER 6

Finding Reliable Information on Coconut Oil the Coconut Oil Weight Loss Secret

Obesity is a major health problem in the US, as well as in many other developed and developing countries. Thus, trying to lose unnecessary weight is an important health concern. Reducing one's weight can have a major impact on quality of life and overall health as obesity or being overweight can lead to a high number of serious health problems including type 2 diabetes, sleep apnea, various cancers (including those of the breast, colon and endometrium), heart attacks, strokes, and hypertension, destruction of joint cartilage, as well as some mental health problems. (It has been observed that there is a link between obesity, depression, decreased cognitive abilities, as well as potentially other mental health problems.)

Therefore, the issue of excessive weight gain should be dealt with seriously, but in a thoughtful and reasonable manner. Losing weight quickly or in the wrong way can have serious health consequences. Thus, it should be said that there is no coconut oil weight loss "secret." Simply following the latest weight loss trend is rarely a good idea. As stated above, one study in Malaysia and one in Brazil did show some loss of waist circumference among some of the obese participants. But it should also be noted that coconut oil is an oil and has lots of fat, albeit relatively healthy, medium chain fatty acids. Therefore, moderation is needed when taking this oil. Weight loss should be a healthy endeavor.

It has been repeatedly stated by health professionals that in order to lose weight and keep it off, you must eat a balanced diet, get regular exercise and get enough sleep daily. These are general guidelines which do not take into account the specific issues that a person who is trying to lose weight might face. So besides losing weight you should also lose it in a way that is best for your body and situation. For example, even after getting enough sleep, eating a balanced diet and getting regular exercise, some people may still have trouble losing weight due to a chemical imbalance within their bodies like an underactive thyroid. Problems with weight loss may even stem from some type of emotional problem like stress. Or a combination of factors may make weight loss difficult.

Additionally, there is the issue of the stage of life you are in when trying to lose weight. Eating a balanced diet, getting regular exercise and sleeping enough sound simple, but what does it mean, especially since the diet, exercise and sleep needs of a person may change based on their age, lifestyle, other health conditions or other factors. In other words, eat a balanced diet can mean different things to different people. For instance, the food preferences and needs of an adult age 75 may be different from an adult aged 25. The sleep needs may differ as well since typically the older you get, the less sleep you need. Additionally, the type of physical activity that you may do as a young person may differ from what you can do as an older adult. Therefore, a weight loss plan needs to take into account your age, gender (women typically require less calories than men), your level of fitness, what sort of health conditions you may have, among other things. This is another reason that simply following a health trend is not a good idea.

So when trying to lose weight and live a healthier lifestyle, how can you get the right information? The most obvious answer is a good place to start: talk to your doctor about your weight loss goals. Depending on your doctor's level of expertise regarding weight loss and your specific health needs, she or he may recommend that you talk to a specialist like a nutritionist, a registered dietician, an endocrinologist or even a psychologist. There are many reasons why a person gains weight and therefore, there can be a myriad of ways in which to deal with reducing your weight.

Along with talking to your doctor about weight loss, you may want to consult other resources, especially if you are interested in weight loss without taking medications. Reliable resources on natural health include the website for the National Center for Complementary and Integrative Medicine which discusses what complementary or alternative medicine is and the types of therapies that have been studied. Much of the information is directed at a lay audience. For health professionals, there are copies of abstracts with more details on the research studies of complementary methods of weight loss. Additionally, the NIH website also contains information on dietary supplements at its Office of Dietary Supplements pages and information about herbal medicine and other alternative treatments on it Medline Plus pages. Another helpful resource for alternative medicine is drugs.com. The website lists various medications, including vitamins, their uses, side effects and possible interactions with other medications or foods. There are also stores which specifically sell natural therapies which stem from health traditions outside the US. For instance, in Chicago, there is the Merz Apothocary which carries various health and beauty products from around the world, such as comfrey root which has been studied and shown to help those with back pain, as well as ankle and knee pain from arthritis. Other trusted sources of information about natural remedies or health supplements include WebMD and medidinenet.com.

CONCLUSION

It is hoped that by reading this information the reader comes away with the understanding little research has been conducted on coconut oil. Therefore, it currently cannot be said that including coconut oil in your diet would lead to weight loss, although the few studies that have been conducted seem to indicate that there might be some benefit for those who are obese. Regardless, coconut oil should be used in moderation. It is, after all, an oil and therefore contains lots of fat. Nevertheless, coconut oil has been used for thousands of years by various cultures around the world for a reason, but more research is needed to determine the exact health benefits that can be gleaned from it.

To hear about Jessica's new books first (and to be notified when there are free promotions), sign up to her New Release Mailing List.

Finally, if you enjoyed this book, please take the time to share your thoughts and post a review on Amazon. It'd be greatly appreciated!

Thank you and good luck!

REFERENCES:

1.Amen, D. G. (2013, August 3). 19 Best Brain Superfoods. [Video file]. Retrieved March 11, 2015 from http://www.amenclinics.com/blog/19-best-brain-superfoods/

2. Tran, M. (2014, January 2). Obesity soars to 'alarming' levels in developing countries. The Guardian. Retrieved from http://www.theguardian.com/us

3. Amen, D.G. The Amen Clinic Method. [Video file]. Retrieved from http://www.amenclinics.com/the-science/see-the-process/

4. Centers for Disease Control. (2011). Obesity. Retrieved March 11, 2015 from http://www.cdc.gov/chronicdisease/resources/publications/AAG/obesity.htm

5. Mayo Clinic Staff. (2012). Hypothyroidism. Retrieved March 6, 2015 from http://www.mayoclinic.org/diseases-conditions/hypothyroidism/basics/definition/con-20021179

6. Zeratsky, K. (2012, August 14). Can coconut oil help me lose weight? Retrieved March 11, 2015 from http://www.mayoclinic.org/healthy-living/weight-loss/expert-answers/coconut-oil-and-weight-loss/faq-20058081

7. Coconut Oil May Decrease Your Waistline . . . if You're a Malaysian Male. Retrieved March 11, 2015 from http://www.uaf.edu/chc/natural-health/COCONUT-OIL-MAY-DECREASE-YOUR-WAISTLINE-1.pdf

8. Liau, K.M., Lee, Y.Y., Chen, C.K., Rasool, A. H.G. (2011). An Open-Label Pilot Study to Assess the Efficacy and Safety of Virgin Coconut Oil in Reducing Visceral Adiposity. ISRN Pharmacology 2011. Retrieved from http://dx.doi.org/10.5402%2F2011%2F949686

9. Mercola, J. (2009, June 2). What Research Really Says about Apple Cider Vinegar. [Video file]. Retrieved from http://articles.mercola.com/sites/articles/archive/2009/06/02/apple-cider-vinegar-hype.aspx

10. (2009, September14, updated November 20, 2009). Retrieved from http://allrecipes.com/cook/coconutgirl/blogentry.aspx?postid=124184

11. Lukuku, J. (2014, August 15). Coconut Oil London Fog. Retrieved March 11, 2015 from http://www.yummly.com/recipe/external/Coconut-Oil-London-Fog-983444

12. Klecker, H. (2013, April 16). Superfood Candy Cups. Retrieved March 11, 2015 from http://www.yummly.com/recipe/Superfood-Candy-Cups-930869?columns=3&position=25%2F58

13. McKenzie, M. (2012, April 12). Banana bread with coffee + coconut oil. Retrieved March 11, 2015 from http://www.yummly.com/recipe/external/Banana-bread-with-coffee-_-coconut-oil-328790

14. Shilhavy, S. (2010, March 19). Roast Chicken with Coconut Oil. Retrieved March 11, 2015 from http://www.yummly.com/recipe/Roast-Chicken-with-Coconut-Oil-1008086?columns=3&position=10%2F58

15. (2011, April 30). Healthy Key Lime Pie Milkshake. Retrieved March 11, 2015 from http://www.yummly.com/recipe/external/Healthy-key-lime-pie-milkshake-325387

16. Amsterdam, E. (2010, April 16). Strawberry Lime Shake. Retrieved March 11, 2015 from http://www.yummly.com/recipe/external/Strawberry-lime-shake-345465

17. Coconut Mango Banana Smoothie Gluten-Free, Vegan Refined Sugar Free. Retrieved March 11, 2015 from http://www.yummly.com/recipe/external/Coconut-Mango-Banana-Smoothie-Gluten-free_-Vegan-_-Refined-Sugar-free-931220

18. Joker Juice Smoothies. Retrieved March 11, 2015 from http://www.food.com/recipe/joker-juice-smoothies-455338

19. Heaping Tablespoon. Retrieved March 11, 2015 from http://www.ask.com/food/heaping-tablespoon-be779fc79424b8e6

20. Baird, M. Double Matcha Green Tea Blast. Retrieved March 11, 2015 from http://www.yummly.com/recipe/external/Double-Matcha-Green-Tea-Blast-996348

21. Murray, K. (2013, December 5). A Hot Cocoa That's Exploding With Superfoods. Retrieved March 11, 2015 from http://www.yummly.com/recipe/external/A-Hot-Cocoa-That_s-Exploding-With-Superfoods_-965195

22. (2014, November 17). Keto Pumpkin Spiced Latte. Retrieved March 11, 2015 from http://www.yummly.com/recipe/external/Keto-Pumpkin-Spiced-Latte-793324

23. Hussong, K. (2015, January 26). Retrieved March 11, 2015 from http://www.yummly.com/recipe/Hot-Chocolate-Zen-992742?columns=4&position=68%2F69

24. Mesa, H. 50/50 Olive Oil/Coconut Oil Blend Healthy Chicken Stir Fry Recipe. Retrieved March 11, 2015 from http://www.foodnetwork.com/recipes/herb-mesa/5050-olive-oilcoconut-oil-blend-healthy-chicken-stir-fry-recipe.html

25. Arneson, B. Salmon with Coconut Sauce. Retrieved March 11, 2015 from http://www.cookingchanneltv.com/recipes/bal-arneson/salmon-with-coconut-sauce.html

26. Tam, M. (2011, February 11). Super Easy Tandoori Chicken. Retrieved March 11, 2015 from http://www.yummly.com/recipe/Super-Easy-Tandoori-Chicken-1003979?columns=4&position=9%2F58

27. (2014, July 10). Paleo Coconut Chicken. Retrieved March 11, 2015 from http://www.yummly.com/recipe/external/Paleo-Coconut-Chicken-992287\

28. (2014, June 29). Coconut Oil Chocolate Chip Cookies. Retrieved March 11, 2015 from http://www.yummly.com/recipe/external/Coconut-Oil-Chocolate-Chip-Cookies-633618

29. (2014, August 9). Blueberry Muffins with Flax Meal and Coconut Oil. Retrieved March 11, 2015 from http://www.yummly.com/recipe/external/Blueberry-Muffins-with-Flax-meal-and-coconut-oil-982997

30. Emmerich, M. (2014, January 9). Coconut Flour Bread. Retrieved March 11, 2015 from http://www.yummly.com/recipe/external/Coconut-Flour-Bread-983476

31. Nevin, K.G., Rajamojan, T. (2004). Beneficial effects of virgin coconut oil on lipid parameters and in vitro LDL oxidation. Clinical Biochemistry. 37(9) 830-5. Retrieved from http://www.sciencedirect.com/science/article/pii/S0009912004001201

32. Assunção, M.L., Ferreira, H.S., dos Santos, A.F., Cabral, C.R., Florêncio, T.M.M.T. (2009). Effects of Dietary Coconut Oil on the Biochemical and Anthropometric Profiles of Women Presenting Abdominal Obesity. Lipids. 44(7) 593-601. Retrieved from http://link.springer.com/article/10.1007%2Fs11745-009-3306-6

33. Intahphuak, S., Khonsung, P., Panthong, A. (2010). Anti-inflammatory, analgesic, and antipyretic activities of virgin coconut oil. Pharmaceutical Biology. 48(2)151-7. Retrieved from http://www.ncbi.nlm.nih.gov/pubmed/20645831

34. Yeap, S.K., Beh, B.K., Ali, N.M., Yusof, H.M., Ho, W.Y., Koh, S.P.,. . . Long, K. (2015). Antistress and antioxidant effects of virgin coconut oil in vivo. Experimental and Therapeutic Medicine. 9(1), 39-42. Retrieved from http://www.ncbi.nlm.nih.gov/pmc/articles/PMC4247320/

35. Shinohara., H., Fukumitsu, H., Seko, A., Fukuwara, S. (2013). Medium-chain fatty acid-containing dietary oil alleviates the depression-like behavior in mice exposed to stress due to chronic forced swimming. Journal of Functional Foods. 5(2), 601-6. Retrieved from http://www.ncbi.nlm.nih.gov/pmc/articles/PMC4247320/#b1-etm-09-01-0039

36. Law, K.S., Azman, N., Omar, E.A., Musa, M.Y., Yusoff, N.M., Sulaiman, S.A., Hussain, N.H.N. (2014). The effects of virgin coconut oil (VCO) as supplementation on quality of life (QOL) among breast cancer patients. Lipids in Health and Disease. 13(1)139. Retrieved from http://www.ncbi.nlm.nih.gov/pmc/articles/PMC4176590/

37. Sun, C.Q., O'Connor, C.J., Roberton, A. M. (2003). Antibacterial actions of fatty acids and monoglycerides against Helicobacter pylori. FEMS Immunology and Medical Microbiology. 36 9-17. Retrieved from http://femsim.oxfordjournals.org/content/36/1-2/9.long

38. WebMD. (2015). Coconut Oil. Retrieved March 9, 2015 from http://www.webmd.com/vitamins-supplements/ingredientmono-1092-COCONUT%20OIL.aspx?activeIngredientId=1092&activeIngredientName=COCONUT%20OIL

39. Jackson, E. From whence come coconuts? The Panama News 12(16). Retrieved March 11, 2015 from http://www.thepanamanews.com/pn/v_12/issue_16/science_01.html

40. The Library of Congress. (2015). Is a coconut a fruit, nut or seed? Retrieved March 11, 2015 from http://www.loc.gov/rr/scitech/mysteries/coconut.html

41. Florida Gardener.com. (2008, June 12). Plant of the Month: Cocos Nucifera-Coconut Palm. Retrieved March 11, 2015 from http://www.floridagardener.com/palms/coconutpalm.htm

42. Bailey, C.C. (2010, February 18). Garden Tips: Are palm trees really a tree, or just a very large plant? Retrieved March 11, 2015 from http://www.tcpalm.com/lifestyle/are-palm-trees-really-a-tree-or-just-a-very

43. United States Department of Agriculture. (2015). Cocos Nucifera L. Coconut Palm. Retrieved March 11, 2015 from http://plants.usda.gov/core/profile?symbol=CONU

44. Tropical Traditions. (2015). What is Virgin Coconut Oil? Retrieved March 11, 2015 from http://tropicaltraditions.com/what_is_virgin_coconut_oil.htm

45. Jalonick, M.C. (2013, November 7, updated 2014, January 23). FDA to Ban Trans Fats. Huffington Post. Retrieved March 11, 2015 from http://www.huffingtonpost.com/2013/11/07/fda-ban-trans-fats_n_4232871.html

46. WebMD. (2015). Lauric Acid. Retrieved March 11, 2015 from http://www.webmd.com/vitamins-supplements/ingredientmono-1138-LAURIC%20ACID.aspx?activeIngredientId=1138&activeIngredientName=LAURIC%20ACID

47. HerbCrust (2013, June 28). Dr. Oz reveals the benefits of Coconut Oil. [Video file]. Retrieved from March 11, 2015 https://www.youtube.com/watch?v=Y3tf3mQiNXI

48. ProYoung Cellular Nutrition. (2014, August 13). Dr. Oz-Coconut Oil Benefits. [Video file]. Retrieved March 11, 2015 from https://www.youtube.com/watch?v=9IhDfMuytR8

49. Rele, A.S., Mohile, R.B. (2003). Effect of mineral oil, sunflower oil and coconut oil on prevention of hair damage. Journal of Cosmetic Science. 54(2)175-92. Retrieved from http://www.ncbi.nlm.nih.gov/pubmed/12715094

50. Centers for Disease Control and Prevention. (2010). Parasites-Scabies. Retrieved March 11, 2015 from http://www.cdc.gov/parasites/scabies/

51. Medical Health Guide. (2011). Coconut. Retrieved from http://www.medicalhealthguide.com/articles/coconut.htm

52. Rudrappa. U. (2015). Coconut Nutrition Facts. Retrieved March 11, 2015 from http://www.nutrition-and-you.com/coconut.html

53. Ruprappa U., (2015). Coconut Oil Nutrition Facts. Retrieved March 11, 2015 from http://www.nutrition-and-you.com/Coconut-oil.html

54. United States Department of Agriculture. (2015). Basic Report: 04047, Oil, Coconut. Retrieved March 11, 2015 from http://ndb.nal.usda.gov/ndb/foods/show/636?fgcd=&manu=&lfacet=&format=&count=&max=35&offset=&sort=&qlookup=coconut+oil

55. Maps of the World. (2015). Top Ten Coconut Producing Countries. Retrieved March 11, 2015 http://www.mapsofworld.com/world-top-ten/world-map-coconut-production-countries.html

56. Das, S. (2015). Symbolism in Hindu Rituals & Worship. Retrieved March 11, 2015 from http://hinduism.about.com/od/artculture/a/symbolism_rituals.htm

57. Schweitzer, V.S. (2006). The Coconut Tree Staff of Life? Retrieved March 11, 2015 http://www.coffeetimes.com/coconut.htm

58. Kapoor, A. (2013, June 12). Importance and Significance of Coconut. Retrieved March 11, 2015. http://panchtatwatloc.blogspot.in/2013/06/importance-and-significance-of-coconut.html

59. Drugs.com. (2015). What is pyridoxine? Retrieved March 11, 2015, from http://www.drugs.com/mtm/pyridoxine.html

60. Felix (2008, July 20). Handmade Coconut Oil-Trini Style. Retrieved March 11, 2015 from http://www.simplytrinicooking.com/2008/07/homemade-coconut-oil-trini-style.html#axzz3TSSTdqEN

61. Make Coconut Not Fat. (2014, April 1) Swedish Chocolate balls using coconut oil recipe. [video file]. https://www.youtube.com/watch?v=DttaRqZizq0

62. Chocolate Banana Wonderful Breakfast Smoothie. Retrieved March 11, 2015 from http://www.yummly.com/recipe/external/Chocolate-Banana-Wonderland-Breakfast-Smoothie-900556

63. Merz Apothocary. (2015) In the Press. Retrieved from http://www.smallflower.com/press/index.cfm

64. National Center for Complementary and Integrative Health. (2015). PubMed Dietary Supplement Subset. Retrieved March 11, 2015 from http://ods.od.nih.gov/Research/PubMed_Dietary_Supplement_Subset.aspx

65. Centers for Disease Control and Prevention (2011). Obesity: Halting the Epidemic by Making Health Easier. Retrieved from http://www.cdc.gov/chronicdisease/resources/publications/AAG/obesity.htm

66. Manning, J. (2014, June 9). 6 Reasons Why You're Gaining Weight. Retrieved March 11, 2015 from http://www.webmd.com/diet/weight-gain-reasons

67. National Sleep Foundation. (2015). How Much Sleep Do We Really Need? Retrieved from http://sleepfoundation.org/how-sleep-works/how-much-sleep-do-we-really-need

MORE BOOKS ON FOOD, HEALTH AND WELLNESS

Click here to check out the rest of Jessica's books on Amazon.

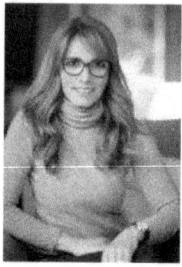

Below you'll find some of my other popular books that are popular on Amazon and Kindle as well. Simply click on the links below to check them out. Alternatively, you can visit my author page on Amazon to see other work done by me.

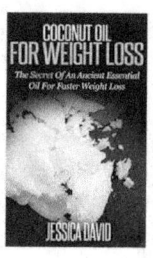 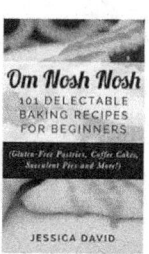 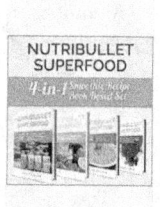 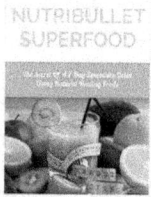 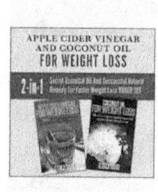

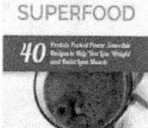 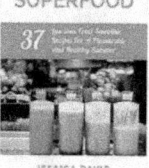 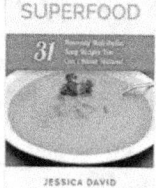 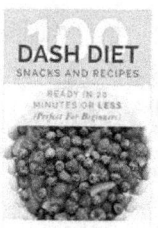 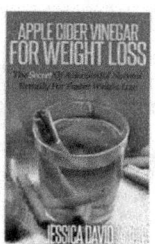

Nutribullet Superfood: 31 Heavenly Nutribullet Soup Recipes You Can't Blend Without

Nutribullet Superfood: The Secret Of A 7 Day Smoothies Detox Using Natural Healing Foods

Nutribullet Superfood: 40 Protein Packed Power Smoothie Recipes To Help You Lose Weight And Build Lean Muscle (Includes: Bonus Protein Add-Ins Guide)

Nutribullet Superfood: 37 Luscious Fruit Smoothie Recipes For A Pleasurable And Healthy Summer

Nutribullet Superfood: 4-in-1 Smoothie Recipe Book Boxed Set

Dash Diet: 100 Dash Diet Snacks And Recipes: Ready In 20 Minutes Or Less (Perfect For Beginners)

Om Nosh Nosh: 101 Delectable Baking Recipes For Beginners (Gluten-Free Pastries, Coffee Cakes, Succulent Pies And More!)

Apple Cider Vinegar For Weight Loss: The Secret Of A Successful Natural Remedy For Faster Weight Loss

Coconut Oil For Weight Loss: The Secret Of An Ancient Essential Oil For Faster Weight Loss

Apple Cider Vinegar and Coconut Oil for Weight Loss: 2-in-1 Secret Essential Oil And Successful Natural Remedy For Faster Weight Loss Boxed Set

Baby Powder: 17 Impressive Uses for Baby Powder You've Never Considered

If the links do not work, for whatever reason, you can simply search for these titles on the Amazon website to find them.